T0143608

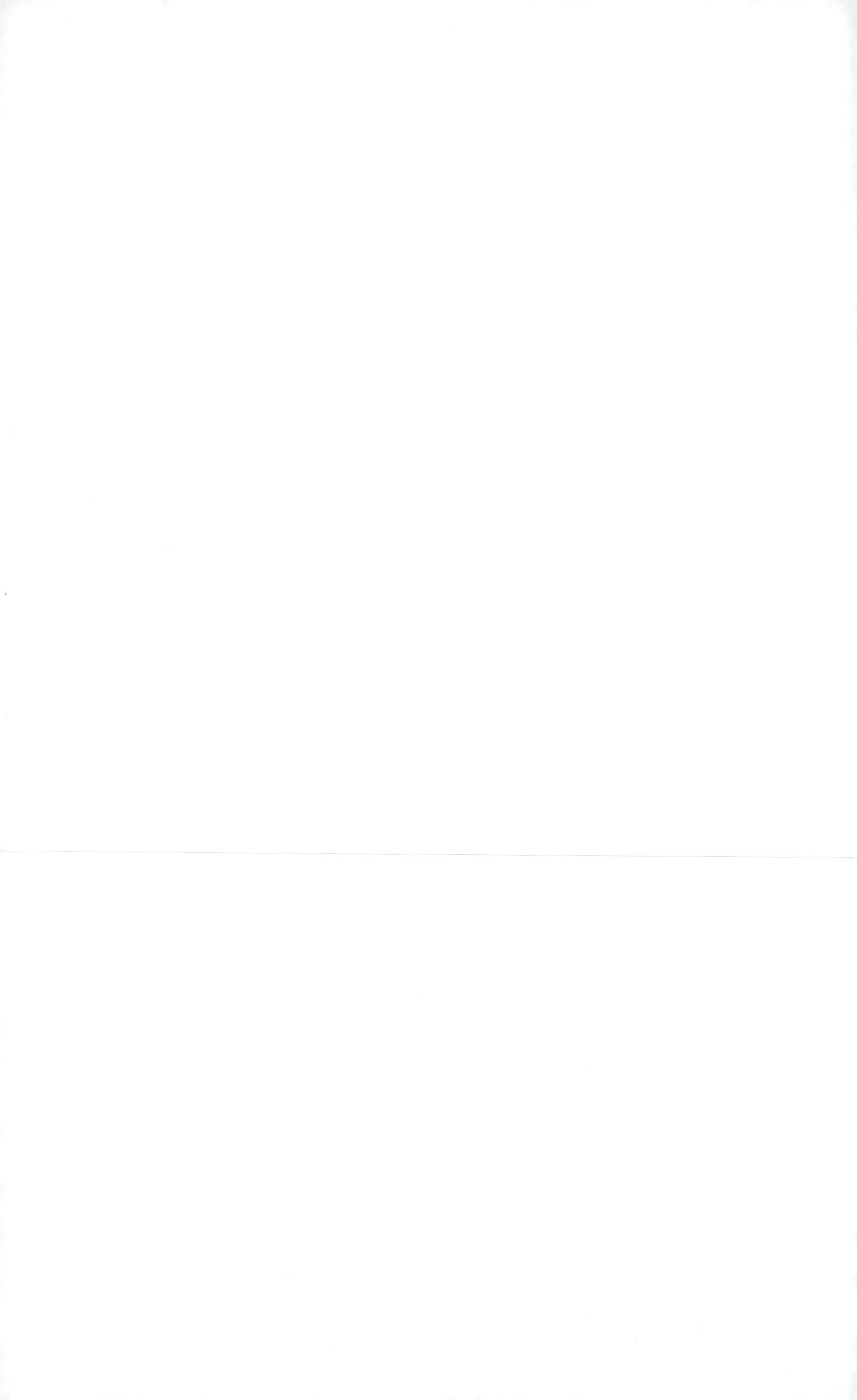

VISUAL TRACKING IN CONVENTIONAL MINIMALLY INVASIVE SURGERY

VISUAL TRACKING IN CONVENTIONAL MINIMALLY INVASIVE SURGERY

SHAHRAM PAYANDEH
SIMON FRASER UNIVERSITY
BURNABY, CANADA

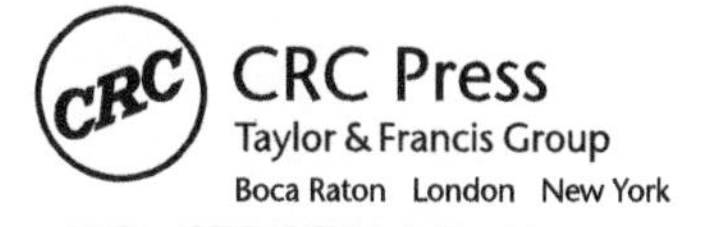

CRC Press is an imprint of the
Taylor & Francis Group, an **informa** business
A CHAPMAN & HALL BOOK

CRC Press
Taylor & Francis Group
6000 Broken Sound Parkway NW, Suite 300
Boca Raton, FL 33487-2742

Printed by CPI on sustainably sourced paper
Version Date: 20160714

International Standard Book Number-13: 978-1-4987-6395-0 (Hardback)

Library of Congress Cataloging-in-Publication Data

Names: Payandeh, Shahram, 1957- author.
Title: Visual tracking in conventional minimally invasive surgery / Shahram Payandeh.
Description: Boca Raton : Taylor & Francis, 2017. | Includes bibliographical references and index.
Identifiers: LCCN 2016022118 | ISBN 9781498763950
Subjects: LCSH: Surgical instruments and apparatus--Design and construction.
Classification: LCC RD71 .P39 2017 | DDC 617.9/178--dc23
LC record available at https://lccn.loc.gov/2016022118

Visit the Taylor & Francis Web site at
http://www.taylorandfrancis.com

and the CRC Press Web site at
http://www.crcpress.com

Contents

Summary

Conventional minimally invasive surgery, which includes laparoscopic surgery, has become commonplace in repairing or replacing tissues and organs within the cavity of the body. This is done by making small incisions, through which an endoscope and long surgical tools are fed in order to reach the inside of the body cavity. By viewing images of the surgical scene on a monitor, the surgeon is able to perform various surgical procedures. The basis of this conventional surgical procedure, which has remained unchanged, is being practiced all over the globe, from the richest nations to the less privileged ones. The procedure is generally performed by one main surgeon and an assistant surgeon, who is responsible for holding and navigating the endoscope. To master this type of surgical procedure one needs to have a certain degree of hand–eye coordination and dexterity. This level of expertise can usually be gained through various virtual or physical training environments. Over the past few years, various degrees of automation have also been introduced in order to assist the surgeon in performing such operations. These can range from a full telerobotic setup to the more conventional designs of surgeon–computer interfaces. The key aspects of developing automation can range from the capability of visually tracking the surgical tools during the operation or training period to tracking a specific landmark located on the surgical scene. These tracking capabilities are particularly important for conventional surgical cases in which economic factors prohibit health providers from deploying telerobotic surgical systems. As such, any automation during the surgical procedure must be done through the image processing of the surgical scene obtained through an endoscope, which is the theme of this book.

The purpose of this book is to introduce the various tools and methodologies that can be utilized to enhance a conventional surgical setup with some degree of automation. The main focus of this book is on the methods for tracking surgical tools and how they can be used to assist the surgeon during the surgical operation. Various notions associated with surgeon–computer interfaces and image-guided navigation are explored with a range of experimental results.

The book starts with some basic motivations for minimally invasive surgery and states the various distinctions between robotic and nonrobotic (conventional) versions of this procedure. Common components of this type of operation are presented with a review of the literature addressing the automation aspects of such a setup. Calibration of the endoscope and its distortion model is presented next. Tracking results of the surgical tool are divided into two classes: marker-based and markerless. The concept of marker-based tracking is that a specially designed barcode added to a surgical tool can be used both to track and identify the tool. Examples of the tracking results are shown for both motion and gesture recognition of surgical tools, which can be used as part of the surgeon–computer interface. In the case of markerless tracking, in which no special visual markers can be added to the surgical tools, the tracking results are divided into two types of methodology, depending on the nature and the estimate of the visual noise. Details of the tracking methods are presented using standard Kalman filters and particle filters. The last chapter of this book is devoted to the approaches that can be utilized for tracking a region on the surgical scene defined by the surgeon. Examples of how these tracking approaches can be used as part of image-guided navigation are demonstrated. Here, using the surgical tool as a 3-D mouse, a region on the surgical scene can be defined and then tracked in the video frames. On this tracked region, for example, information such as medical images or graphical data can be overlaid and repositioned based on the spatial tracking information of the marked region.

Shahram Payandeh, PhD, P.Eng.
Simon Fraser University
Burnaby, British Columbia, Canada

CHAPTER 1

Overview of Minimally Invasive Surgery

There have been many definitions associated with the term *minimally invasive surgery* (MIS). We state here the most common definition, which is also directly related to the theme of this book. MIS is a procedure in which a surgeon can access the surgical site through small incisions or natural openings into the body. In general, through one of these ports of entry the surgeon inserts a long-stem endoscope with an illuminating tip that allows the viewing of the surgical site on an overhead monitor. Through other ports of entry, various long-stem surgical tools are inserted that allow the surgeon to perform manual surgical procedures. In general and from the patient's perspective, this type of surgical procedure results in a reduction in hospital stay, a faster recovery time, less chance of infection, and a reduction in large tissue scars when compared with open surgery. Currently, MIS is performed in a large number of general surgical procedures for the gallbladder, lungs, heart, spine, and urinary system (Singla et al. 2009). The surgical tools and systems used for a typical MIS procedure in an operating room are very similar (Figure 1.1). For example, cholecystectomy (i.e., gall bladder removal), one of the most common MIS procedures, is performed using laparoscopy (Sages 2016).

Laparoscopic surgery as a minimally invasive technique was successfully introduced for gynecological procedures in the early 1970s (Spaner and Warnock 2009). Nowadays, more and more surgical procedures are likely to be performed using laparoscopic techniques as the advantages of

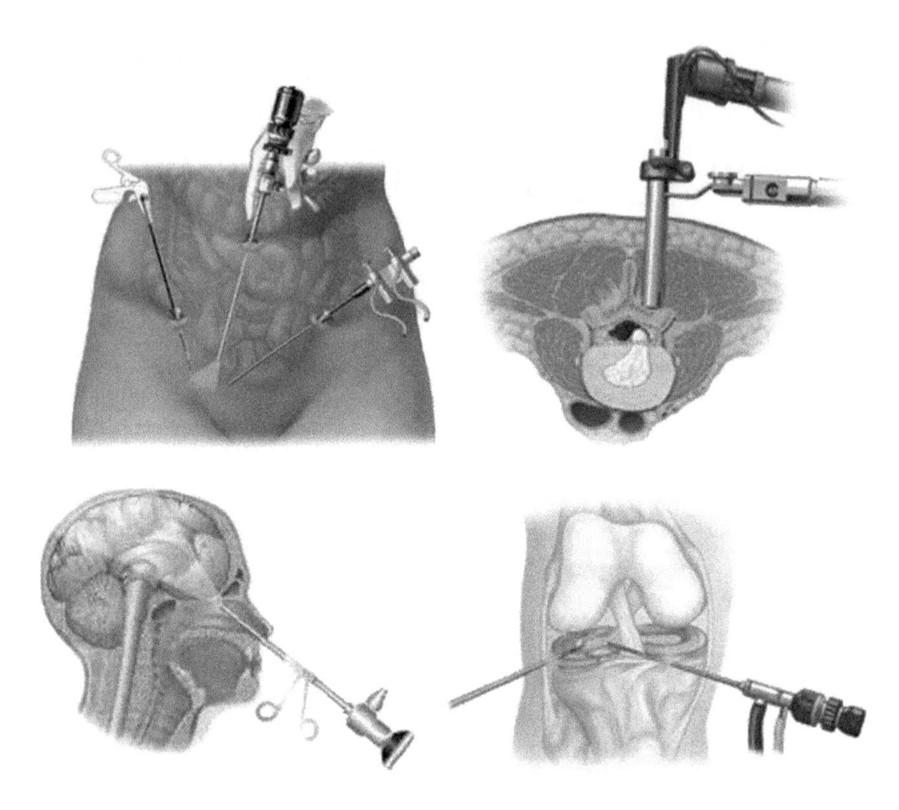

FIGURE 1.1 Placement of the endoscope in various MIS procedures.

minimally invasive procedures are further realized. In laparoscopic surgery, a surgical operation is performed with an endoscope (laparoscope) and a number of long, thin, rigid instruments (see Figure 1.2) inserted into the body through several small incisions created by the surgeon. As stated, when compared with traditional open surgery, it can provide less pain, faster recovery, and smaller scars from the incision points. During conventional two-handed laparoscopic procedures, the field of view of the surgical site through an endoscope sometimes needs to be adjusted. This adjustment is usually accomplished by the surgeon's assistant, who holds the endoscope while viewing the surgical site and listening to the verbal commands of the surgeon.

A common surgical challenge in conventional laparoscopic surgery is the lack of 3-D perception of the surgical site given in a conventional operating room theater. The surgeon needs to view the surgical site through a single camera (which can have more than one charged-couple device [CCD] sensor for better resolution) that can offer a clear 2-D projection of

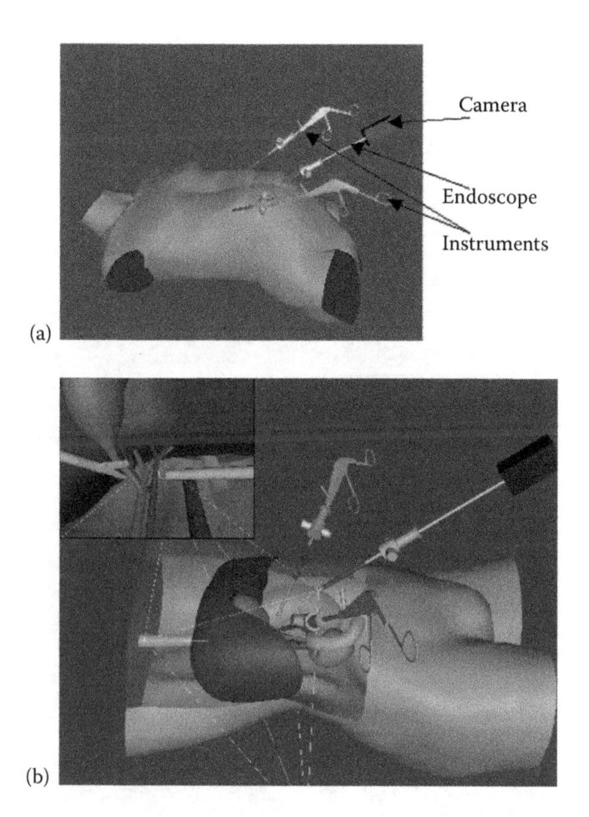

FIGURE 1.2 Visualization of the main instruments used for laparoscopic procedures: (a) placements of the laparoscope and surgical tools; (b) endoscopic view of the surgical site.

the surgical site (Figure 1.3). Currently, technologies are being introduced for creating a stereo view of the surgical site (Visionsense 2016). However, in general, the implementation of such tools requires the surgeon to wear a headpiece, which results in a loss of peripheral vision. Besides the main requirement of viewing the surgical site on the overhead monitor, the surgeon also wants to have a clear view of the other tools, equipment, and personnel around the operating table. In addition, the benefits of 3-D imaging in comparison with conventional 2-D imaging are not highly valued as yet in the medical communities (Clinical 2016).

Besides MIS having a number of benefits for patients, it also presents additional challenges for surgeons. These include the loss of a direct view of the surgical site, the loss of tactile perception, and unnatural hand–eye coordination. To compound such challenges, a direct view of the surgical site is replaced by a distorted endoscopic view and the surgeon is

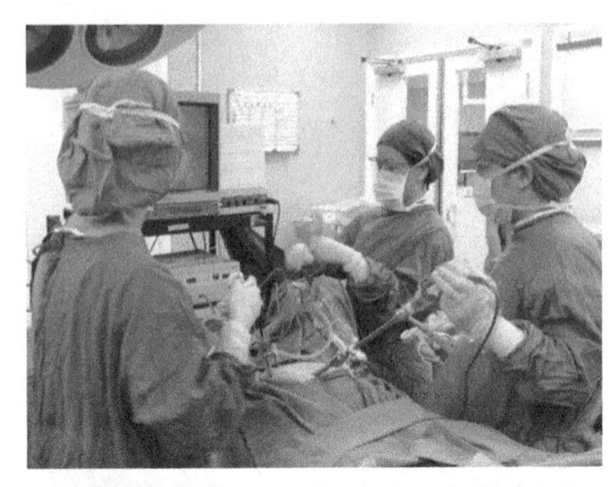

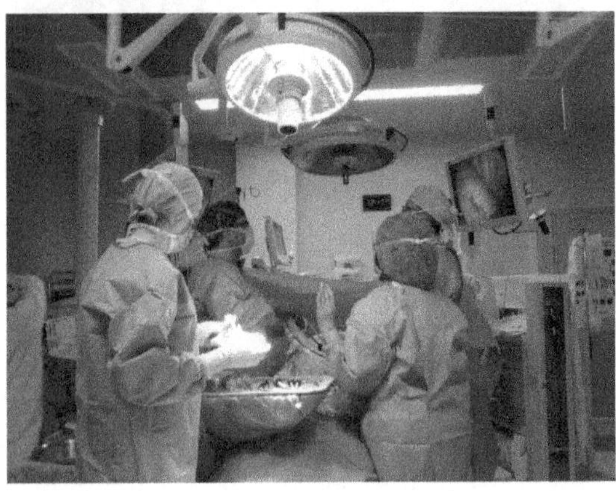

FIGURE 1.3 Two examples of a conventional operating room setup for MIS.

required to manipulate the surgical site using long-stem surgical instruments. Surgeons have to operate by looking at viewing monitors displaying images of cavities at awkward angles with a very restricted range of views. Moreover, they can no longer touch tissues with their hands, as only long, thin surgical instruments small enough to go through the tiny incision holes are used. Therefore, surgeons have to develop new hand–eye coordination and instrument manipulation skills in order to cope with the less ergonomic operating environment and limited working space.

In performing a conventional MIS procedure (Figure 1.3), a typical surgical theater consists of the surgeon, the assistant to the surgeon, who holds and positions the endoscope, and the supporting nurses, who supply surgical instruments and medical information about the patient. Historically, besides some of the challenges in performing MIS previously stated, the introduction of some degree of automation in such procedures has been desirable. This can lead to a reduction in the number of surgical personnel in the operating room and also may result in a consistent view of the surgical site through the endoscope. Some of the earlier attempts to introduce some degree of automation are presented in Faraz and Payandeh (1998, 2000). Full automation was later introduced through a product by Intuitive Surgical in 2000 (Intuitive 2000). The main idea of this product is to replace the presence of the surgeon and, during various intervals, the presence of supporting personnel in the operating theater, and to have robotic arms holding the endoscope and surgical instruments. These robots are controlled by a surgeon located at a remote workstation (usually in the operating room). By viewing 3-D images of the surgical site on the surgical workstation and by manipulating special hand-held mechanisms, the surgeon can control the viewing angle and motion of the surgical tools at the site.

OVERVIEW OF MINIMALLY INVASIVE SURGERY TRAINING ENVIRONMENTS

Mastering the challenges in performing MIS procedures requires the surgeon to enhance his or her skills by both using training environments and by performing the actual procedures under the supervision of an experienced surgeon. The training environments range from an emulated physical setup consisting of an endoscope and surgical tools inserted inside a training box to a virtual surgical training environment. In the virtual environment, the view of the endoscope and the presence of the surgical tools are represented graphically. The position of the endoscope in the virtual environment can be controlled externally and the trainee can interact with the virtual surgical tools through various user interface devices (Payandeh and Li 2003; Payandeh 2015; LapMentor 2016).

Virtual training environments can offer a variety of learning scenarios with varying degrees of difficulty. Since both the motion of the surgical tools and their interaction with the virtual environment are computed and displayed through various algorithms, it is also possible to collect such data for further analysis and evaluation. As such, various metrics can be developed that can be used to assess the performance of the trainee.

One of the drawbacks of deploying such a system is its initial cost and the further costs associated with its maintenance. Besides offering a platform for mastering the basic hand–eye coordination that is needed for a general class of MIS (Shi and Payandeh 2010), the virtual simulation environment also lacks the necessary realism. In order to increase the realism of the virtual surgical site, numerical methods and associated material properties of tissue and organs need to be collected and modeled.

Surgical training boxes are another alternative for enhancing the basic skills needed for MIS. They offer a physical *in vitro* setup in which the body cavity is recreated as a box using basic materials such as rubber or plastics. An endoscope is inserted inside the box through an opening and, depending on the type of surgical procedure, surgical tools are inserted

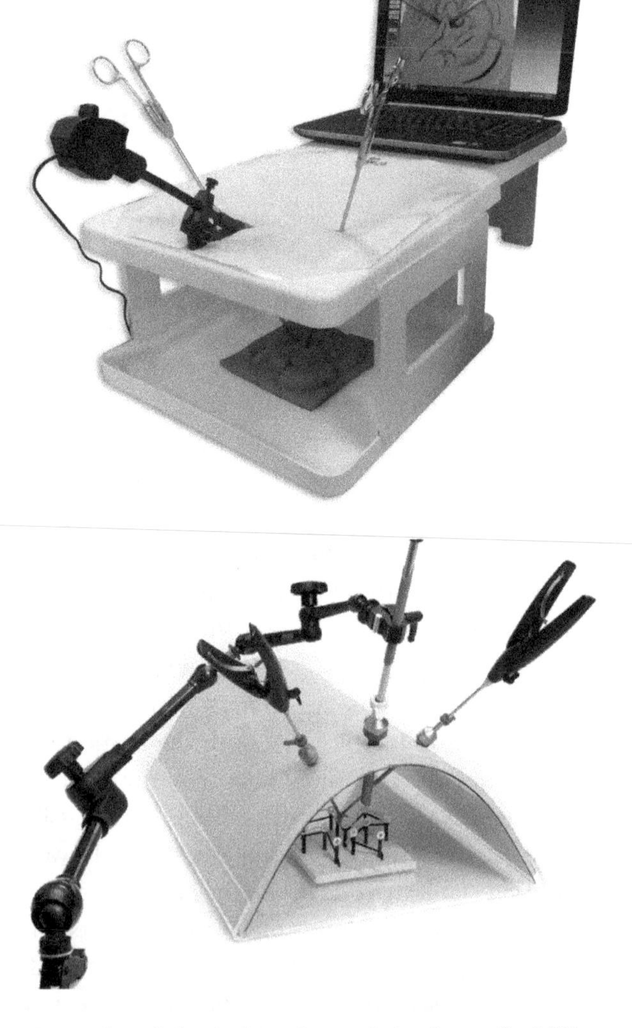

FIGURE 1.4 Examples of physical *in vitro* training boxes for MIS.

through various predefined incisions (Figure 1.4) (LapTrainer 2016; Fls 2016; Seal 2016).

Some of the key advantages of surgical training boxes are the ease of their manufacturability and their cost-effectiveness. They can be assembled using off-the-shelf materials and are being utilized in most surgical curricula around the world (Ma and Ujiki 2015). However, while offering a physical setup that can be used to emulate the actual surgical environment, these types of training boxes do not offer any degree of automation. For example, being able to visually track the surgical tool during a basic surgical procedure can offer a metric for evaluating the performance of the surgical residence. Tracking of the surgical tool combined with the task duration can offer another type of metric that can be used as part of the performance skills assessment. In addition, enhancing such basic surgical training boxes with advanced notions of visual mentoring and guidance can further increase their range of effectiveness. For example, by monitoring the motion of the surgical tools during a specific procedure, graphical images and overlaid information can be displayed that can be used as a mentoring tool during image-guided navigation (Parada and Payandeh 2009). The visual tracking methods presented in this book can be used as one of the main frameworks for the further enhancement of such physical surgical training environments with some degree of automation.

CONVENTIONAL VERSUS ROBOT-ASSISTED MINIMALLY INVASIVE SURGERY

Conventional MIS is performed in most countries around the world regardless of their financial and economic status. Besides the usual costs associated with using an operating theater, the costs related to surgical theater setups for conventional MIS are nominal (JHN 2015). Similar to automating other application areas, introducing some degree of automation to the surgical field and in particular to MIS can offer both advantages and disadvantages. One of the main disadvantages of introducing a high degree of automation through a teleoperation system (Intuitive 2000) is the initial high cost of its deployment and the associated maintenance costs. As a result, such systems are only available to medical centers and institutions around the world in better financial positions and with more means. In addition, since the deployment of robot-assisted surgery, various studies have been conducted to further understand its overall advantages to health care when compared with the conventional approaches to performing MIS.

As a part of the comparative studies, Sarlos et al. (2012) concluded that robot-assisted laparoscopic hysterectomy and conventional laparoscopy compare well in most surgical aspects, but the robotic procedure is associated with longer operating times. The postoperative quality-of-life index was better. However, in the long term, there was no difference, and subjective postoperative parameters such as analgesic use and return to activity showed no significant difference between groups. Another study conducted by Baek et al. (2012) concluded that robot-assisted surgery is more expensive than laparoscopic surgery for rectal cancer. Considering that robotic surgery can be applied more easily for low-lying cancers, the cost-effectiveness of robotic rectal cancer surgery should be assessed based on oncologic outcomes and functional results from future studies. Wright et al. (2013) analyzed the uptake of robotically assisted hysterectomy to determine the association between the use of robotic surgery and rates of abdominal and laparoscopic hysterectomy, and compared the in-house complications of robotically assisted hysterectomy with abdominal and laparoscopic procedures. They concluded that between 2007 and 2010, the use of robotically assisted hysterectomy for benign gynecologic disorders increased substantially. Robotically assisted and laparoscopic hysterectomy had similar morbidity profiles, but the use of robotic technology resulted in substantially higher costs.

In general, the most common drawback to introducing an advanced degree of automation to surgical procedures is the associated cost. Although the advancement and availability of tools and technology can result in an overall cost reduction for deploying surgical robots, there also exist some challenges in reassuring their safe integration, design, and usage. For example, the BBC (2015) reported that robotic surgery had been linked to 144 deaths in the United States.

MOTIVATIONS AND OBJECTIVES OF THIS BOOK

This book explores various approaches in which it is possible to introduce some level of automation to the conventional MIS and surgical training environments. The framework is based on utilizing the existing tools that are present in a conventional operating room, which include an endoscope, surgical tools, and a camera system. The images from the camera used on the viewing monitor are also captured and processed using a conventional computational platform (e.g., a desktop personal computer). As explored in this book, by being able to track the motion and orientation of surgical tools, it is possible to achieve various implementations of the notions related to a surgeon–computer interface (SCI). In this paradigm, similar to the notion of a computer mouse as a human–computer interface, the tracked motion of the surgical tool can be used as a surgical mouse. Using the calibration parameters of the endoscope, this analogy can further be extended to a 3-D mouse paradigm, where the spatially tracked information of the surgical tool can be utilized. This allows the surgeon, as needed, to retrieve and interact with medical information related to the patient through overlaid graphical images (i.e., augmented reality). For example, Figure 1.5 shows a conceptual representation of an operating theater where, by using a surgical tool, the surgeon is making a particular gesture. Through visual recognition of the gesture, it is possible for the computer to retrieve medical images and display the information on an overhead monitor, which can be used to guide the surgeon in a particular surgical procedure. Besides the automatic retrieval of information, the proposed framework of this book offers approaches that can be further extended to allow surgeons to manipulate the overlaid graphical images on their endoscopic display to further register them on the surgical site. Preoperative image registration on the surgical site to assist with image-guided surgery has been a challenging task. The method of this book is to offer approaches in which, using surgical tools, the surgeon can manually position overlaid preoperative graphical images on the surgical site. In addition, it shows that it is possible to introduce the notion of image tracking to track endoscopic features on the surgical site. As such, it is possible to register preoperative graphical information on the endoscopic

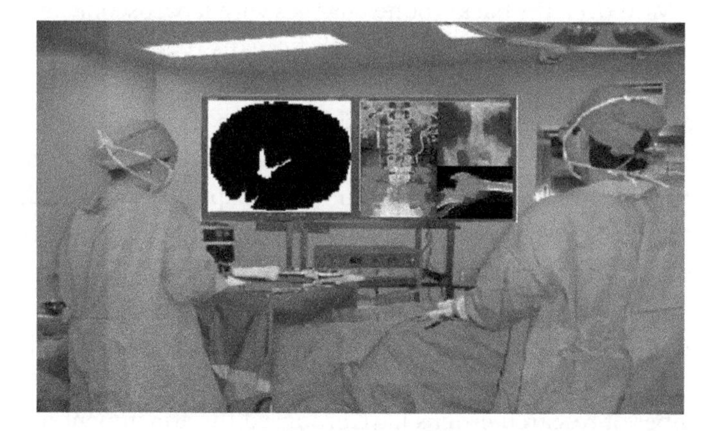

FIGURE 1.5 A conceptual operating room, where the gesture of the surgical tool is recognized (left monitor) and then associated with certain medical images (right monitor).

site and maintain its position regardless of the motion of the endoscope. This allows surgeons to also place virtual overlaid markers on the surgical site using their tools and to anchor them to the tissue regardless of the motion of the endoscope.

LITERATURE OVERVIEW

In this book, the methods for tracking surgical tools are divided into two main categories. The first category is the tracking methodology, where the surgical tools are designed with specific artificial visual markers and gestures located on the tool. The second category is the general case, where surgical tools do not have any specific markers assigned to them and their shapes are used to accomplish visual tracking results. The last chapter of the book explores and presents some results that can be used for tracking special features on the surgical scene.

Surgical tool gesture recognition is easier than human hand gesture recognition as surgical tools have a fixed color and shape. Their surface colors do not differ from one another, as human skin tones do. Furthermore, surgical tools do not deform, as human hands do. In other words, the number of variations of one marked surgical tool gesture is less than that of a human hand gesture. However, surgical tool gesture recognition presents its own unique challenges, the most difficult being extracting surgical tools from the background. In most human hand gesture recognition literature, the background is often very simple and constant. In our case, the background, which is composed of body tissues and organs, is more complex. Moreover, the background changes with laparoscopic movement and the reflections from body tissues and organs further complicate the surgical tool extraction process.

In order to achieve an accurate position of the surgical tool, a number of challenges must be overcome. One is that the only available measured information is through the use of video signals captured by the endoscope. Another challenge is the complexity of the surgical scene, which contains blood, vessels, organs, and deforming tissue. Reflections can be a problem for tracking when using metallic instruments. Occlusion, an unstable background, and the presence of smoke can also increase the difficulty of surgical tool tracking.

A number of research groups have proposed the attachment of specific markers on the surgical instrument in order to facilitate the visual tracking task. Wei and Arbter (1997) and Tonet et al. (2007) rely on color information to facilitate visual tracking by stamping the surgical tool with a color marker. To avoid sterilization issues, a biocompatible color marker is used by Bouarfa et al. (2012) to detect and track instruments in laparoscopic video. Loukas (2013) has explored the results of color-based surgical tool tracking in AR interaction with an emulated laparoscopic training box. In some earlier works, color strips on the surgical instrument are regarded as fiducial markers to help with tracking (Zhang et al. 2002). Instead of using color information, some groups apply optical techniques in their visual tracking. In the robot-based tracking method presented by Krupa et al. (2003), a light-emitting device is placed on the tip of the tool that can project laser dots onto the surface of organs. Based on the projected optical marker, the system is able to locate the instrument on the screen. A similar application of optical markers has been developed by Shin et al. (2010).

Instead of using a marker, some utilize segmentation techniques and detection to assist with the visual tracking of surgical tools. A fast segmentation algorithm of gray regions in color images has been proposed for tracking gray or metallic instruments (Doignon et al. 2005). This method is based on a joint hue–saturation color feature. Cano et al. (2008) use an edge detector to segment the input image and detect the tip position of the tool by means of color analysis. Similar to the work of Doignon et al. (2005), Ryu et al. (2013) first segment the image into organ area and instrument area by *k*-means clustering according to their color signatures and then apply a chain of image-processing techniques, such as Canny edge detection (Canny 1986), binarization, and morphology, to extract the instrument from the background. Based on the assumption that the surgical instruments mostly have straight-line structures, a combination of the Hough line transform and the conditional density propagation algorithm is employed in tool tracking (Climent and Hexsel 2012). To obtain a more efficient and accurate tracking performance, Reiter et al. (2012) have designed a feature descriptor to help with tracking. This feature descriptor contains information such as color value, spatial derivatives, gradient magnitude, and orientation, making the instrument more distinctive.

Tracking systems are used to determine the position of the target in image-guided procedures. Different approaches to visual tracking have been proposed to solve increasingly complex and diverse tracking conditions, especially for multiple target tracking. In general, the tracking approaches can be categorized into bottom-up and top-down procedures. The bottom-up procedure is to localize and track the target for each independent image sequence. The position of a target is located by extracting characteristics such as edges, corners, and colors from the image sequences. In a tracking scenario, an *object* can be defined as anything that is of interest for further analysis. For example, points or centroids (Zhang and Payandeh 2002; Salajegheh 2008), primitive geometric shapes (Comaniciu et al. 2003) (rectangles, triangles, ellipses, etc.), silhouettes and contours (Davis 2001), and more complex articulated shape models (Rehg and Kanada 1995) can also be considered objects.

Selecting the right features plays a critical role in tracking. In general, the most desirable property of a visual feature is its uniqueness, so that it can be easily distinguished from the feature space. For example, color is used as a feature for histogram-based appearance representations. As stated, a robust color-tracking method is presented in Tonet et al. (2007), using the hue, saturation, and value (HSV) color mode. In general, color-based tracking is fast, especially for multiple targets. The main drawback is its lack of robustness and stability in cases of variant illumination and partial occlusion. Another problem is that it requires artificial color coding on the target. Unlike color-based approaches, contour-based tracking is reliable and can cope with partial occlusion and light variance. Algorithms that track the boundaries of objects usually use edges as the representative feature, since edges usually generate strong changes in image intensity. The most popular is the Canny edge detector. There are other visual tracking approaches based on motion detection. One method uses frame differences to create a motion history image (MHI) that represents a function of the recent motion in a sequence (Bradski and Davis 2002). By analyzing the motion, the orientation and velocity of the moving target can be extracted.

All of the bottom-up approaches shown extract a set of features from each frame (typically boundary-like and corner-like features) and then attempt to establish correspondences between the sets of features. However, the drawback of this approach is its inability to deal with multiple moving targets in a cluttered and complex environment. The algorithm often fails to label each of the targets—for example, two sets of surgical tools.

A different approach for video tracking is the top-down process, where filtering and data association are taken into consideration. Not only is the target tracked based on its salient features (such as edge, color blob, and shape), but prior information about the object is also involved, dealing with object dynamics and evaluating different hypotheses (such as the constant velocity of the object in motion). The computational complexity for these algorithms is usually much higher due to matrix operation and probability-based computation. However, it is more practical in a cluttered environment where multiple targets are being tracked. The system is represented using a state-space model, where the state is predicted based on the system model or estimated based on observation. The approach is recursive in nature and operates in two phases: prediction and update. Each state is first propagated according to the system model (prediction stage), then corrected in terms of the observations (update stage). Gaussian probabilistic trackers such as the Kalman filter (KF) (Dellaert and Thorpe 1997; Fu and Han 2012) address the general problem of trying to estimate the state of a discrete-time process that is governed by a linear stochastic difference equation. As expectation for more realistic visual tracking grows, more versatile and advanced nonlinear and non-Gaussian elements are desirable in order to model the underlying system more accurately. Nonlinear trackers, such as particle filters (PFs), are therefore being explored (Nummiaro et al. 2003; Arulampalam et al. 2002).

All top-down methods need an initialization process, requiring the first target position. Moreover, the observation needs to be generated from the camera sensor each frame to update the system model. Therefore, the filter cannot work without cooperating with feature-based detection or motion analysis. In this, we explore an approach that combines both advantages, forming a hybrid system. This system consists of bottom-up feature detection and top-down Kalman filtering, supporting multitarget tracking in a noisy environment.

For both marker-based and markerless tracking methods, the information from a static image is not enough to obtain a reliable result. Instead, the information contained in a sequence of images should be taken into account to improve the accuracy of the tracking. Namely, the tracking results from the previous frames must be considered. To estimate the position of the surgical tool, in this book some Gaussian probability-based estimators, such as the KF, extended Kalman filter (EKF), and PF, are introduced to the tracking system. As stated, these estimators are usually composed of two phases: predication and correction. The tracking problem is converted into the state of the process needing to be estimated. The state is first predicted according to a system model and further corrected by real-time observation. The application of the estimation step can return more accurate and reliable tracking results. In particular, the KF has been widely used for tracking in a linear dynamic system with Gaussian densities (Bouarfa et al. 2012; Loukas 2013; Ryu et al. 2013; Sa-Ing et al. 2011). In this book, a feature-based KF tracking module was developed to track the position of the surgical tool. In addition, an EKF was developed to tackle cases where the dynamic and observation models are nonlinear but where the noise is additive and Gaussian (Reiter et al. 2012; Huang et al. 2013). The advantage of deploying a PF framework for visual tracking is its less restricted assumptions on the expected dynamics of the motion, so that it does not rely on any linear and Gaussian assumptions associated with the tracking problem and can deal with more complex scenarios (Mckenna et al. 2005; Speidel et al. 2006).

To provide intraoperative guidance in MIS and its relevant training with AR technology, a robust region-tracking algorithm is necessary to maintain the connection between virtual object and real scene regardless of endoscope motion. As distinct from tracking a surgical tool, where one can rely on color distribution or structured features such its edges and its rigid shape to distinguish the target from the background, region tracking in surgical scenarios is often more challenging. One problem is the deformable tissue structures inside the target region. This increases the complexity of the target content. Furthermore, the color distribution of the target region is usually similar to its surroundings, so that traditional color analysis is not suitable. To cope with these difficulties, there are two types of tracking strategies: feature based and model based.

In feature-based tracking methods, the target region is represented and tracked in the feature space. A discriminative and repeatable feature description (SIFT, SURF, BRIEF, STAR, etc.) is required to depict local structures according to the information from the spatial neighborhood. The feature representation is invariant to changes in viewing conditions such as scale, orientation, and contrast. By matching the feature descriptors from different images, the same region can be detected according to the correspondence.

An integrated framework for tissue tracking under stereo cameras is presented by Yip et al. (2012). The salient features in the surgical scene are extracted using a combination of the STAR feature detector and BRIEF descriptor. A densely populated map of tissue deformation in 3-D space is generated from these features. Stoyanov et al. (2004) developed a real-time feature-based semidense spatial reconstruction method for laparoscopic applications. Feature matching is first conducted across stereo image pairs and then applied to propagate the surface structure into neighborhood image regions. Giannarou et al. (2013) proposed a probabilistic framework utilizing an affine-invariant anisotropic feature detector and an EKF for region tracking in MIS. After generating an initial 3-D surface feature map from SIFT descriptors, an EKF framework is responsible for estimating the current stereo camera motion and 3-D surface feature location relying on 2-D BRIEF descriptors. This system is able to provide persistent surface tracking in real time.

For the model-based tracking methods, the target region is considered a template. According to a deformable model, the correspondence between the pixels in the template and those in a new incoming image can be found. A biomechanical model of tissue deformation combined with image constraints is proposed for intraoperative guidance in MIS (Pratt et al. 2010). Stoyanov et al. (2004) integrated their salient feature-tracking approach with a constrained geometrical model to achieve robustness to occlusion and specular highlights (Stoyanov and Yang 2009). In the work of Gaschler et al. (2010), the epipolar constraints are incorporated into sum-of-square differences (SSD) minimization to deal with affine region tracking in stereoscopic MIS. To assist the surgeon during minimally invasive cardiac surgery, a state motion model is designed to estimate the moving partition of the heart's surface (Bader et al. 2007). Similarly, an affine motion model was employed to help the tracking of natural landmarks on the heart surface for beating-heart surgery (Ortmaier et al. 2005).

LAYOUT OF THE BOOK

The book is organized as follows: Chapter 2 presents an overview of tools that have been used in performing conventional MIS. These basic tools range from endoscopes and cameras to various surgical instruments. Due to the wide-angle lens system used in the conventional design of endoscopes, the endoscopic views of the surgical site are usually distorted. In order to create linear relationships in the image plane, this chapter presents a method for creating an undistorted image model from the raw images of the endoscopic lens system. Some of the methods for visual tracking in this book rely on the optical parameters of the endoscopic lens system. This chapter also presents an approach for calibrating and computing optical parameters such as the focal length. Chapter 3 presents some approaches, based on conventional surgical tools, to designing a marker-based surgical tool tracking system. This chapter also presents how surgical tools can be used as part of a tooltip gesture recognition system, which can be used as part of the overall SCI system. Here, marked gestures made by the tip of the surgical tool are used as artificial markers that are made by the surgeon at various instances during the operation. A collection of these marked gestures can be stored and compared with various other gestures that the surgeon makes during the surgery. A recognized gesture can then be associated with a specific action as a part of the SCI. Chapter 4 presents what is referred to as a *markerless* surgical tool tracking system. In comparison with Chapter 3, the need to design and place (or configure) a specific marker on the tool is eliminated. The approach of this chapter utilizes various image-preprocessing methods in order to segment surgical tools from their background and utilizes the KF framework to track the predefined state associated with the segmented images. The underlying assumption for such a framework is based on the Gaussian distributions of noise and state being within their nominal values. Chapter 5 presents methods for tracking surgical tools when a non-Gaussian distribution of nominal values of the state of the tool is utilized. The method is based on PF estimation, where the initial state of the segmented tool is used to propagate the probable state of the tool in the next time instant. The predicted state is then obtained using the weighted average of all the propagated states. This chapter also presents the results of a hybrid approach, where a probabilistic tool segmentation method is combined with the PF framework. Chapter 6 presents tracking results where, instead of tracking surgical tools for designing an SCI environment, the selected scene on the surgical site is tracked. Experimental studies have shown that by tracking a predefined region of interest, a graphical object can be augmented in the live video stream, which can be used in the context of image-guided navigation and surgery.

SUMMARY

MIS has a number of key advantages for patients. In addition, the approach offers some key challenges to the surgeon performing such procedures. Conventional nonrobotic setups for performing such procedures do not offer any degree of automation in comparison with more complex and expensive robotic versions. In conventional procedures that are practiced all around the world and in countries with varying degrees of financial status, basic tools such as endoscopes, surgical tools, and camera viewing systems are used. The objective of this book is to explore several approaches, guided by the notion of visual tracking, that can be used to introduce automation and information retrieval, both during surgery and at various stages of training.

CHAPTER 2

Endoscope Setup and Calibration

THIS CHAPTER PRESENTS AN overview of surgical tools and systems that are used in a conventional minimally invasive surgical procedure. For example, basic tools that are used for laparoscopic surgery can include: insufflators, optical systems, lavage aspiration systems, trocars, and surgical tools such as graspers or needle drivers. For visual tracking, one of the most important components of minimally invasive surgery (MIS) is the optical system, which is presented here in more detail in comparison with other surgical tools that are present in a conventional MIS surgical theater.

OPTICAL SYSTEM

The optical system can be divided into three main parts: the light source, the endoscope, and the optical cable responsible for transmitting the light from a light source to the surgical cavity and the camera.

Light Source

There exist two types of sources used in MIS: halogen and xenon. The main difference between them is their color temperatures (5000–5600 K for halogen and 6000–6400 K for xenon). For example, the Karl Storz 615 Xenon Light Source (Storz 2016) is designed to provide the illumination necessary for most endoscopic applications (and is also used as a part of the experimental setup in this book). The xenon lamp color temperature approximates bright sunlight and is considered unmatched for visual and

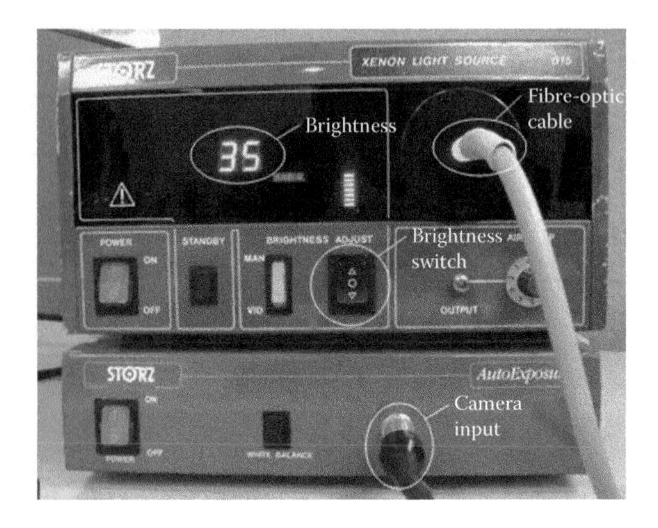

FIGURE 2.1 A typical source of light for endoscopic viewing. The light source is transmitted through a fiber-optic bundle mounted around the endoscope to the surgical site. The light source also allows adjustment of the illumination conditions to be set.

photographic color rendition. Figure 2.1 provides an illustrative description of the light source. When video cameras are used, close-up viewing is hampered when there is too much light, whereas more distant views may be too dark. A typical light source used in MIS has the capability for manual adjustment.

Endoscope and Cables

The cables connected to the endoscope and to the light source are part of the illumination system. When light is transmitted, the cable is responsible for attenuating the light to a lesser or greater extent, depending on its type and especially its condition. Two types of cable are currently available on the market: optic cables and gel cables. Although optical cables are fragile, this type is normally chosen because of its flexibility and lower maintenance (this type of cable is also selected as a part of the experimental setup of this book).

Many types of endoscopes offering various optical properties exist. For example, a Hopkins rod lens endoscope is shown in Figure 2.2 (Storz 2016). Figure 2.2a illustrates how the refraction occurs as light passes through small lenses seated at distant intervals; Figure 2.2b shows how the rod lenses are seated at close intervals, resulting in better light transmission and a reduction in diameter; and Figure 2.2c shows an oblique

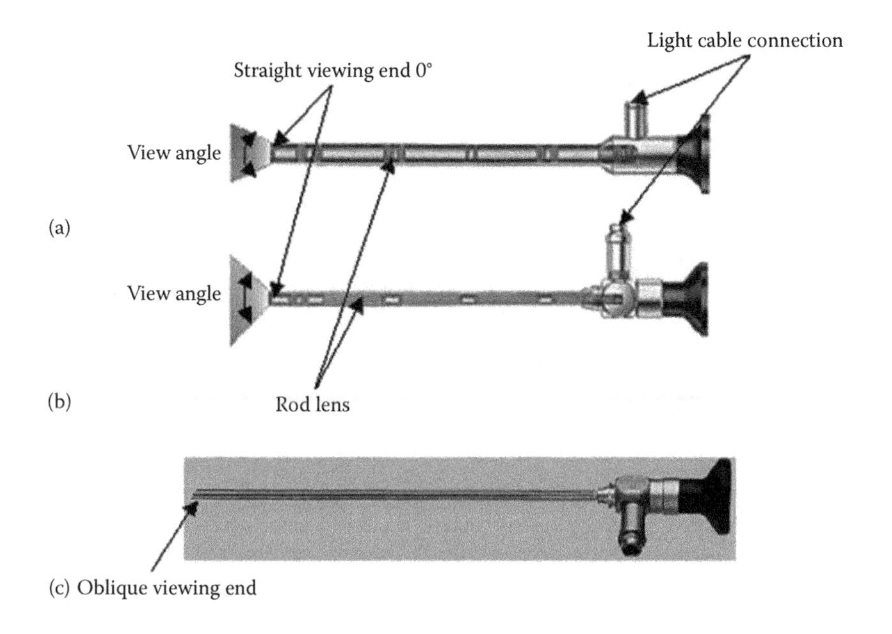

FIGURE 2.2 Example of a rod lens endoscope: (a) an endoscope featuring a conventional lens system; (b) a Hopkins rod lens endoscope; (c) a 45° forward-oblique endoscope.

endoscope. Generally, the oblique angle is designed for 30° or 45°. This type of endoscope is of interest for certain procedures such as viewing the external iliac bifurcation when performing a laparoscopic lymphadenectomy or the laparoscopic treatment of hiatal hernias.

Video Camera

The camera is fitted with charged-couple device (CCD) sensors. These sensors transform the properties of the actual image (photons) into electronic images that can be transmitted to the viewing monitor. For some of the experimental setups, the Karl Storz Supercam is utilized. The Supercam is a small, lightweight, easy-to-operate, high-resolution camera for video monitoring and recording of endoscopic procedures. Later advancement of the video camera system has introduced three CCD high-definition cameras, such as the IMAGE1 camera (Figure 2.3; Storz 2016).

Surgical Tools

Surgical tools are used by a surgeon to assist in performing various remote operations through incisions at the surgical site, including palpation, section, dissection, suturing, destruction, and hemostasis. Typical surgical

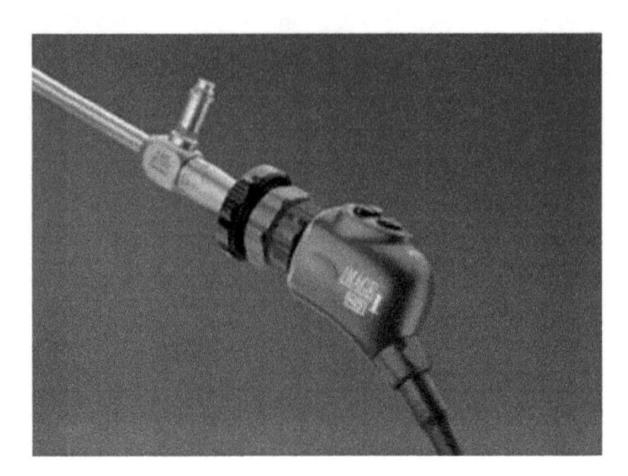

FIGURE 2.3 Karl Storz IMAGE1 SPIES camera with full-HD three-chip configuration. (From Storz, Karls Storz endoscope, https://www.karlstorz.com/ca/en/index.htm, last accessed February 2016.)

tools that are often used include laparoscopic scissors, forceps, dissectors, needle holders, and multipurpose instruments. Typical diameters of these instruments are from 5 to 10 mm (Figure 2.4).

These tools, when passed through an artificial incision point into the body, are passed through another instrument called a trocar. Trocars are important components of MIS with a number of functionalities. For

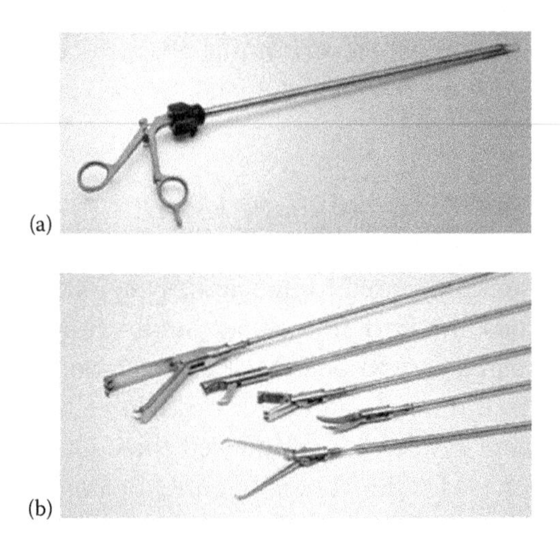

FIGURE 2.4 Example of minimally invasive surgical tools showing (a) the shape of the handle and (b) examples of the surgical tips. (From Ackermann, Ackermann finest surgical technology, http://www.ackermanninstrumente.de/index.html, last accessed February 2016.)

example, for creating an incision point, they are used to guide the blade through the skin, which can be used as a port of entry to the body. They are used to maintain an airtight interface between the surgical tools and the port of entry.

IMAGE PROCESSING

The live video stream from the endoscopic camera can be captured for further processing. If live video streams are in analog format, they need to be digitized for further processing using signal-processing hardware and a computational platform. In general, digitalization comprises three steps: (a) *scanning or digitizing* is the process of sequentially addressing a small area on the video stream; (b) *sampling* is the process for measuring the gray level (or color level) of an image at each pixel location; and (c) *quantization* is the step for representing the measured value by an integer (Tanimoto 2012). These three steps result in a numerical representation of an image from a sample of the video stream.

For example, the digitized image can be represented by a 2-D gray-level matrix. For each location of a pixel at (u,v), its gray level can be associated with $f_{u,v}$. For an image $[F]$ with $n \times m$ pixels, we can write

$$[F] = \begin{bmatrix} f_{0,0} & f_{0,1} & \cdots & f_{0,n-1} \\ f_{1,0} & f_{1,1} & \cdots & f_{1,n-1} \\ \cdots & & & \\ f_{m-1,0} & f_{m-1,1} & \cdots & f_{m-1,n-1} \end{bmatrix} \quad (2.1)$$

Through the application of various operations on input matrix $[F]$, it is possible to manipulate the original image using various image-processing algorithms. For example, grayscale resolution is defined as the number of gray levels per unit of measurement of image gray amplitude. Storing a digital image in 8-bit bytes, for example, yields 256 levels of gray scale. Generally, larger images have a higher grayscale resolution and are more clearer than small images. On the other hand, the computation time that is required for processing the input image also increases.

An efficient data structure is also a key factor that influences the image-processing speed. The commonly used data structures for image processing include 2-D and 1-D matrices. Though the 2-D matrix as a form of data structure is a popular one due to its clear and direct expression, it requires a fixed memory allocation, while using a 1-D matrix in pointer mode enables us to use dynamic allocated memory. A point (u, v) in an m row by n column 2-D matrix can be represented as $(v-1)\times n+u$ in a 1-D matrix. Using pointers to represent this 1-D matrix, we can allocate, delete, and resize memory as needed (GPU units can also be implemented to facilitate the matrix manipulation tasks) (Daga et al. 2011; Liu and Vinter 2014; Shi and Payandeh 2008).

Various techniques for solving visual tracking problems have been proposed. Techniques used for visual tracking can include optical flow, feature point correspondence, edge or contour correspondence, active contour models, and model-based matching. In visual tracking associated with MIS, there also exists a diverse range of instruments with different shapes and sizes that can be inserted into the surgical area with various angles of inclination with respect to the endoscope axis.

Endoscopic Camera Calibration

Defining a relationship for pixel-to-world mapping is known as *camera calibration*. Once the camera has been calibrated, we can transform the image pixel coordinates to their real-world equivalents. Camera calibration is a critical first step in many applications, such as the dimensional measurement of mechanical parts, tracking, camera-on-robot configuration, and robot vehicle guidance. Camera calibration has also been investigated extensively by many researchers—for example, Chen et al. (1995) and Tsai (1987).

In general, endoscopic images have particular characteristics. The endoscopic view angle, typically between 65° and 75° (Figure 2.2), is narrow compared with the wide field of view of the human eye. Thus, vision is limited. To enlarge the field of view, generally, wide-angle lenses are used in endoscopes. However, wide-angle lenses intrinsically have barrel distortion (the transformation of straight lines into curves). Barrel distortion causes the image position to be distorted along radial lines from the image center. This type of distortion is nonlinear: image areas farther away from the center appear significantly smaller. In this section, a calibration method is proposed that assumes the image located within the small center area is free of distortion.

Typical parameters that are used for calibration can be classified into two classes: extrinsic and intrinsic. This section presents methods for determining intrinsic parameters—namely, the effective *focal length*, the *real image center*, and the *scale factor*. Extrinsic parameters, which include rigid body transformation from the world coordinate system to the camera coordinate system, are also discussed.

Figure 2.5 illustrates the basic geometry of the camera model, where (x, y, z) is defined as the world reference coordinate system and (x_c, y_c, z_c) is defined as the camera coordinate system; (x, y, z) also presents the 3-D coordinates of an object P in the world coordinate system, while (x_c, y_c, z_c) is the coordinate of the same point P in the camera coordinate system, with the z_c axis aligned with the optical axis. Here, the camera coordinate frame is defined at the tip of the endoscope. If a perfect pinhole model assumption is used, (x_d, y_d) (not shown in Figure 2.5) is the image coordinates of $P(x_c, y_c, z_c)$ projected into the image plane (Asari et al. 1999). (V_i, V_j) are the coordinates used in the image buffer. Additional scale factors need to be specified that relate the image coordinates in the front image plane to the image buffer coordinate system (Zhang 2002).

The focal length f is the distance between the front image plane center o_c and the optical center o. Here, we define the image center as the optical axis passing through the image plane. In principle, the image center should be the center of the image plane. But in practice, especially in the endoscopic image, the real image center is distorted due to the imperfect grid of the endoscope lens.

In the following, first we propose a simple and fast method to obtain the real image center, then a method for calculating calibration parameters such as the effective focal length and the scale factor. The first problem is how to find the real image center. Since the surgical cavity is dark, an external light source is used for illumination purposes (Figure 2.1).

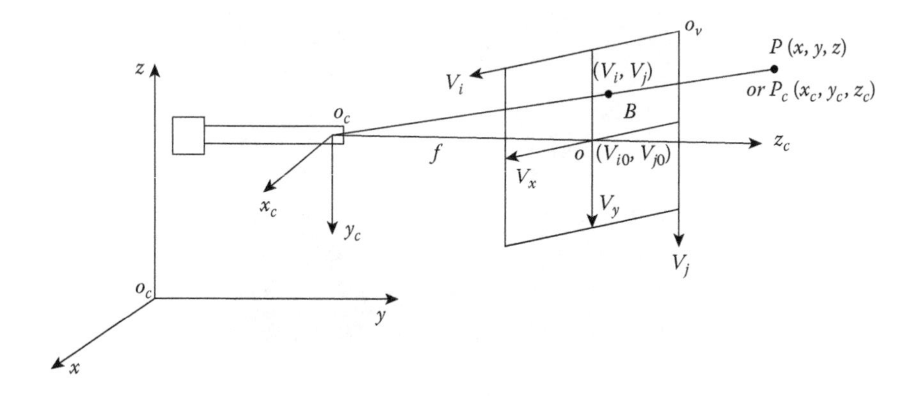

FIGURE 2.5 Camera geometry with perspective projection.

A fiber-optic cable is used to transmit light to the side of the endoscope. The light source is evenly distributed through the rod lens. If we point the endoscope perpendicular to a white background, the light source forms a white circle in the image, as shown in Figure 2.6a.

Inspired by this feature, we find a simple method of locating the real image center is to let the endoscope point to a white background and then capture the image. The center of the white circle in the image is defined as the real image center. The result is shown in Figure 2.6b. Others, such as Asari et al. (1999), consider the distortion in the endoscopic image. They propose using straight-line patterns and selecting the intersection of lines that remain straight in the endoscopic image as the real image center without using any complex calculations.

The second parameter to be calibrated is the real focal length. As shown in Figure 2.5, transforming from 3-D camera coordinates (x_c, y_c, z_c) to image coordinates (V_i, V_j) based on the perspective projection with pin-hole camera geometry, we can write the following equations:

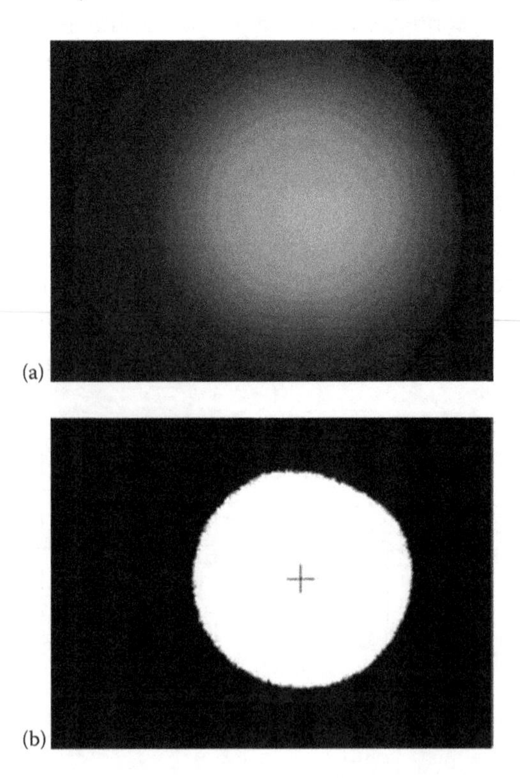

FIGURE 2.6 Endoscopic images: (a) the original grayscale images; (b) the binary image (the center has been marked).

$$\frac{oo_c}{z_c} = \frac{f}{z_c} = \frac{(V_i - V_{i0})S_x}{x_c} = \frac{(V_j - V_{j0})S_y}{y_c}$$
$$x_c = \frac{z_c(V_i - V_{i0})S_x}{f}, \; y_c = \frac{z_c(V_j - V_{j0})S_y}{f} \tag{2.2}$$

where:

oo_c is the distance between the center of the image buffer to the center of the camera coordinate frame

(V_{i0}, V_{j0}) are the row and column numbers of the image center

S_x and S_y are the scale factors that map the real image coordinates (x_d, y_d) of a point P into the image buffer coordinates (V_i, V_j)

When V_i, V_j, X_c, and z_c are known parameters, the effective focal length can be calculated from Equation 2.2. Also, when f, V_i, V_j, x_c, and y_c are known parameters, we can work out the depth information z_c of an object in the field of view.

Scale factors S_x and S_y can be obtained using the following formula:

$$x_d = (V_i - V_{i0})S_x$$
$$y_d = (V_j - V_{j0})S_y \tag{2.3}$$

In general, manufacturers of CCD cameras supply information on the center-to-center distance between adjacent sensor elements in the y direction (i.e., scale factor S_y) as a fixed value:

$$S_y = N_{fy} / d_y$$

where:

N_{fy} is the number of pixels in the y direction

d_y is the dimension of CCD in the y direction

Scale factor S_x is an uncertain value due to a number of reasons, such as slight hardware timing mismatches between the image acquisition hardware and the camera scanning hardware, or imprecision in the timing of the imaging scanning itself. Here we propose a simple and fast method to obtain the relationship between S_x and S_y.

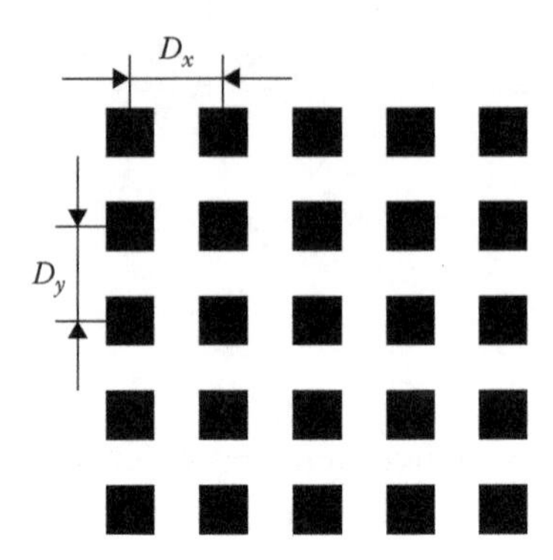

FIGURE 2.7 The pattern image for calibration.

We use the endoscope to capture an image of known dimensions (e.g., square grids), then we compute the center-to-center distances of the squares D_x and D_y, as shown in Figure 2.7, of the pixel unit in the x and y directions, using the equation

$$S_x / S_y = D_x / D_y$$

So

$$S_x = S_y \times D_x / D_y \tag{2.4}$$

In actual implementation, we can measure the center-to-center distances of several squares and use their mean values to reduce the possible error that may be introduced by the image-processing.

Lens Distortion and Correction Methods

No lens can produce perfect images. Common imperfections are aberrations that degrade the quality or sharpness of the image and lens distortions that deteriorate the geometric quality (or positional accuracy) of the image. Endoscopic images have fundamental lens distortion due to the wide-angle design of the objective lens of endoscopes. Wide-angle lenses are used in endoscopes because they provide larger viewing fields. However, lens distortion will result in the erroneous measurement of image positions in the resulting images.

To eliminate the distortion effect, corrections should be applied to measurements of the resulting endoscopic images. Subsequent analysis of laparoscopic images, such as estimating quantitative parameters (area and perimeter), is of considerable importance while performing clinical endoscopy (such as tumor measurement). Unless the distortion is corrected, estimation errors can increase, which can affect various diagnostics or medical procedures (Hatada et al. 1991; Margulies et al. 1994).

Lens distortion is classified as either *radial* or *tangential*. Radial distortion, as its name implies, causes the image position to be distorted along radial lines from the optical axis. Radial distortion includes barrel distortion, pincushion distortion, or a combination of these two types. Tangential distortion is due to imperfect centering of the lens components and other manufacturing defects in a compound lens; it is also called *decentering*—that is, the optical center and the lens are not strictly collinear. The pixel shift is away from the optical center and the new position lies at a new angle location as measured from the optical center. Tangential lens distortions are generally very small and are seldom corrected (Wolf 1983).

To capture a larger field of view in a single endoscopic image, wide-angle lenses are often used—for example, in laparoscopic procedures. Thus, barrel-type radial distortion is common in laparoscopic images due to the wide-angle configuration of the camera lens (see Figure 2.8). Areas further from the center of the field of view appear smaller than they really are. For the reason described previously, in this section we only consider barrel-type distortion.

Three different methods of correcting radial distortion are: (a) determining the required corrections from a radial lens distortion curve, (b) interpolating corrections from a Table lookup, and (c) through computational

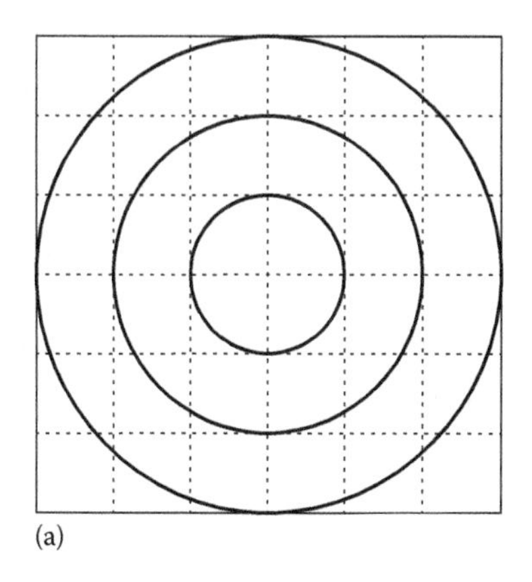

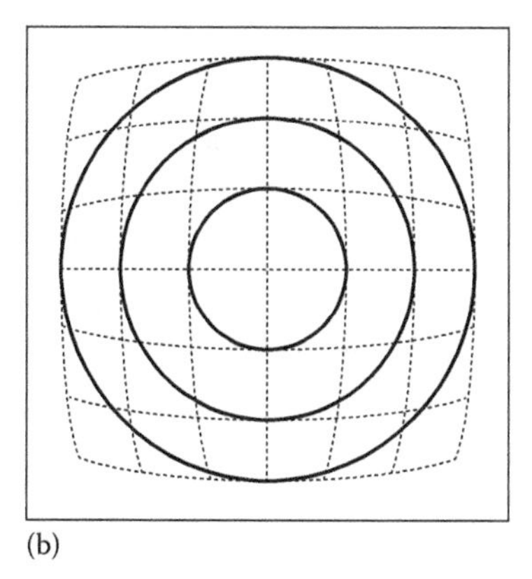

FIGURE 2.8 Barrel-type distortion. (a) Undistorted grid pattern; (b) distorted grid pattern.

procedures in which the radial lens distortion curve is approximated by a polynomial. Here, we have adopted the last method of correcting the lens distortion though polynomial approximation. For this purpose, the least squares method is utilized in order to find the coefficients of the polynomial. Given the polynomial approximation, it is then possible to manipulate the live endoscopic images in order to obtain undistorted ones.

Radial Lens Distortion Model

The radial lens distortion model consists of two image planes. The distorted image plane is represented by (V_i', V_j'), while the distortion correction image plane is represented by (V_i, V_j). Their corresponding centers are represented by (V_{io}', V_{jo}') and (V_{i0}, V_{j0}). The center of the distortion correction image can be chosen arbitrarily. Unlike the method proposed by Smith et al. (1992), who selected these two centers at different locations, here, both centers are selected to be the same as the real image center. That is, the straight lines that pass through this point remain straight in the distorted image plane.

Using the polar coordinate definition of the origin at the real image center, a point P' in the distorted image plane can be represented as

$$\begin{aligned} r' &= \sqrt{(V_i' - V_{i0}')^2 + (V_j' - V_{j0}')^2} \\ \theta &= \arctan\left(\frac{V_j' - V_{j0}'}{V_i' - V_{i0}'}\right) \end{aligned} \tag{2.5}$$

where magnitude r' is the distance of P' to the center (V_{io}', V_{jo}'). The corresponding point P' in the corrected image plane is P. Point P can be represented by polar coordinates (r, θ). Because we assume that the distortion is purely radial, the polar angle is unchanged in the distorted and corrected image planes—hence, $\theta = \theta'$.

The objective of the distortion model is to find the relationship between P and P'. As shown in Figure 2.9, the relationship between r and r' is

$$r' = r + \Delta r \tag{2.6}$$

where Δr can be represented as an odd-ordered polynomial series (Wolf 1983):

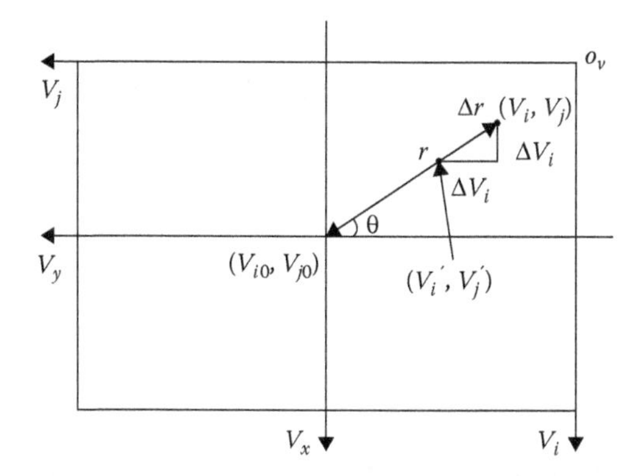

FIGURE 2.9 Components of radial distortion. The image point $P(V_i, V_j)$ is radically displaced by Δr to the new position $P(V_i', V_j')$.

$$\Delta r = k_1 r + k_2 r^3 + k_3 r^5 + k_4 r^7 + \cdots \tag{2.7}$$

where k_i ($i = 1, 2, 3\ldots$) are the expansion coefficients. The reason for using odd-ordered degree-interpolating polynomials is because it has been shown that even-ordered degree-interpolating polynomial filters are space variant with phase distortion (Schafer and Lawrence 1973). This is attributed to the fact that the number of sampling points on each side of the interpolated point always differs by one. As a result, interpolating polynomials of even degrees are not considered.

After obtaining the coefficients, the new pixel location in the corrected image plane can be calculated as $r' = r - \Delta r$ (see Figure 2.9). The relationship can be written as

$$\frac{r}{\Delta r} = \frac{x}{\Delta x} = \frac{y}{\Delta y} \tag{2.8}$$

The new pixel location in terms of the two components (Δx and Δy) can be defined as

$$\begin{aligned} x' &= x - \Delta x = x\left(1 - \frac{\Delta r}{r}\right) = x\left(1 - k_1 - k_2 r^2 - k_3 r^4 - \ldots\right) \\ y' &= y - \Delta y = y\left(1 - \frac{\Delta r}{r}\right) = y\left(1 - k_1 - k_2 r^2 - k_3 r^4 - \ldots\right) \end{aligned} \tag{2.9}$$

An estimate of the coefficient of the polynomial is required as the next step of the process in order to define the polynomial form for mapping a distorted to an undistorted image.

Estimation of Coefficients

The polynomial coefficients define the shape of the curve. They can be calculated by nonlinear regression analysis, such as the least squares method, to obtain a best curve fit to a given data set (obtained from experiments). The calibration pattern (Figure 2.7) is used to obtain the square center positions in the distorted image. Since it is assumed that the distortion is purely radial, it is also assumed the distortion is circularly symmetric. Without loss of generality, testing squares that lie in the horizontal or vertical planes in the image can represent the general distortion pattern for the whole image. For a given data set—for example, $S = \{C_1, C_2, \ldots, C_i, \ldots, C_N\}$—let N be the number of columns of testing squares for each $C_i(r_i, \Delta r_i)$, where r_i represents the radial distance between the center of the square and the real image center, and Δr_i is the distortion at a radial distance r_i. Let us consider the polynomial series of degree $2M + 1$:

$$\Delta r_i = k_0 r_i + k_1 r_i^3 + k_2 r_i^5 + \cdots + k_j r_i^{2j+1} + \cdots, \quad j = 0,1,\ldots,M \tag{2.10}$$

The deviation of a point from its correct image position can be written as

$$F_i = y_i - \sum_{j=0}^{M} k_j r_i^{2j+1} \tag{2.11}$$

The least squares problem is then to find the values of k_j, $j = 0,1, \ldots, M$, so as to minimize

$$\sum_{i=1}^{N} \left[y_i - \left(\sum_{j=0}^{M} k_j r_i^{2j+1} \right) \right]^2 \tag{2.12}$$

where k_j can be calculated from

$$\frac{\partial F_i}{\partial k_j} = 0, \quad for \quad j = 0,1,\ldots,M \tag{2.13}$$

From Equation 2.10, $M+1$ simultaneous equations are obtained, which may be represented in matrix form as

$$AK = Y \tag{2.14}$$

where:

$$A = [r_i^{2j+1}]_{(M+1)\times(M+1)}, \quad \text{for } i = 0,1,\ldots,M,\ j = 0,1,\ldots,M$$
$$K = [k_0, k_1, \ldots, k_M]^T$$
$$Y = [y_0, y_1, \ldots, y_M]^T$$

Equation 2.14 can be computed as

$$K = (A^T A)^{-1} A^T Y \tag{2.15}$$

The matrix K consists of the most probable values for unknowns k_0, k_1, …, k_M. The detailed derivation of K is shown in Appendix I.

Once the expansion coefficients are computed, all pixels from the distorted image are mapped onto the corrected image. However, one issue that needs to be dealt with is the direction of mapping. One approach is mapping from the distorted image plane to the corrected image plane using the following relationship:

$$r = k_1 r' + k_2 r'^3 + k_3 r'^5 + k_4 r'^7 + \cdots \tag{2.16}$$

where r' is the radial distance measured in the distorted image plane and r is the radial distance measured in the corrected image plane. One of the limitations of this approach is that it can result in having blank pixels in the corrected image. This is due to the nonlinear expansion of the image, where the original image is mapped onto a new enlarged one (see Figure 2.10; notice there are many blank pixels in the image, especially in the peripheral part). This problem can be avoided by utilizing

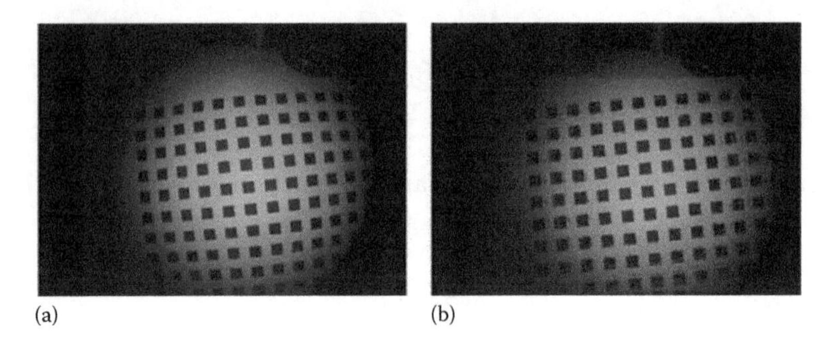

FIGURE 2.10 (a) Original image; (b) the result after distortion correction.

an alternative mapping method—namely, inverse mapping, which is mapping from the corrected image plane to the distorted image plane. The coefficient estimation method described in Equation 2.9 uses the inverse mapping method. In Equation 2.9, r is measured in the corrected image plane. Thus, for every pixel in the corrected image plane, the corresponding location in the distorted image is obtained using the polynomial in Equation 2.9. The information (e.g., gray level) for that pixel location is assigned to the pixel in the corrected image plane. In the case that the pixel positions calculated using the inverse mapping in Equation 2.9 are nonintegers, we simply round it to the closest integer. Because the corrected image enlarges the distorted image with barrel-type radial distortion, it is possible that several pixels in the corrected image may find the same pixel in the original image. In this way, all pixels in the corrected image plane can find their corresponding pixel value, thus generating a complete, undistorted image.

EXPERIMENTAL STUDIES

Experimental studies are carried out in order to evaluate the proposed methods for determining the intrinsic parameters of the endoscope and the associated distortion model. The calibration procedure is conducted to determine the real image center, the scale factors, and the endoscope focal length.

Locating the Real Image Center

Before the experiment, a calibration pattern is used to evaluate the feasibility of the proposed method for locating the real image center. First, we locate the image center and overlay two crossed lines to mark the real image center at their intersection. Second, we place a patterned image

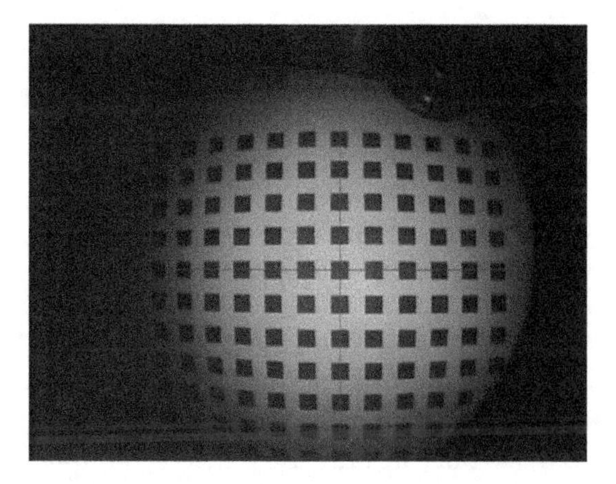

FIGURE 2.11 Sample test image that was used as a part of the proposed image center location.

perpendicular to the optical axis of the endoscope. The pattern image is placed in such a way that one square in the pattern image is aligned with the two overlaid crossed lines (see Figure 2.11). Experimental results show that for one row of squares that lie along one of the overlaid lines, their centers have the same V coordinates (e.g., the second row of Table 2.1). For one column of squares that lies along the overlaid line, their centers have the same V_i coordinates (e.g., the second column of Table 2.1). It can be observed that other columns or rows of squares do not share this feature, which supports the feasibility of the proposed method for locating the image center.

Obtaining Image Coordinates

Here, the centers of squares are selected as the calibration points. Since the objective is the computation of the intrinsic parameters, information regarding a measure of distance between the centers of squares in the world coordinate unit is needed.

The image coordinates for calibration were computed as follows: (a) a grayscale image is acquired (Figure 2.12a), and (b) the threshold image is obtained and the center of each blob are computed (Figure 2.12b).

Computation of the Intrinsic Parameters

Scale factors: Scale factors provide the ratio of a distance on the image to the same distance in the world coordinate unit. Here, we assume the image distortion around the center area is negligible is examined. After

TABLE 2.1 (V_i, V_j) Coordinates of the Center of Calibration Squares around the Overlaid Crossed Lines

(310, 128)	(**360**, 129)	(410, 129)
(309, 176)	(**360**, 176)	(411, 177)
(308, **226**)	(**360**, **226**)	(412, **226**)
(308, 277)	(**360**, 278)	(412, 278)
(309, 327)	(**360**, 328)	(411, 328)

computation of the real image center, the test grid is placed perpendicularly at a distance of 50 mm from the endoscope, with the center of one of the squares located at the real image center (Figure 2.12). To reduce the influence of lens distortion, we only use nine central squares for calculations. As shown in Table 2.2, it is observed that for squares lying in the same row or column, their corresponding V_i or V_j coordinates are off only

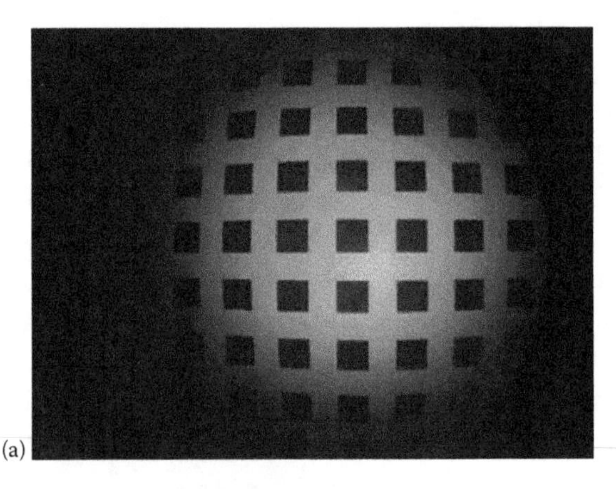

(a)

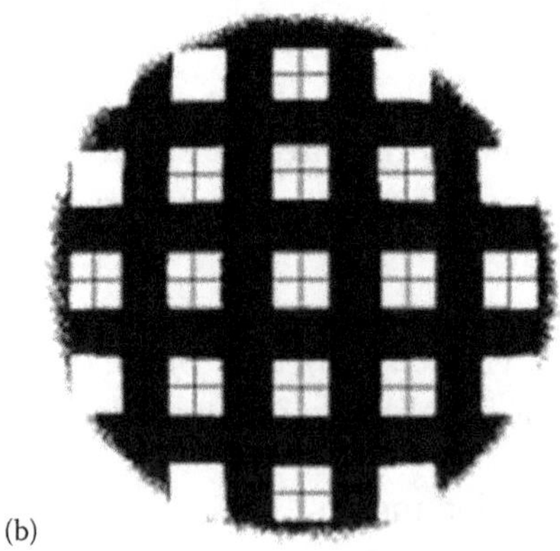

(b)

FIGURE 2.12 Computation of calibration coordinates: (a) the original grayscale image; (b) the binary image with the marked computed centers of blobs.

TABLE 2.2 (V_i, V_j) Coordinates of the Center of Nine Squares in the Central Area (Pixel Unit)

(**298**, 169)	(363, 168)	(430, 169)
(**297**, 234)	(364, 234)	(431, 234)
(**297**, 300)	(363, 301)	(431, 300)

by, at most, 1 pixel (e.g., given the first column in the table, the coordinates of the three points along V_i are 298, 297, 297). We use the mean values of the center-to-center distance between neighbor squares along V_i and V_j to obtain the scale factors ($S_x/S_y = 66.67/65.83 \approx 1$).

Focal length: Data from the previous experiment indicate that the scale factors in directions V_i and V_j are approximately similar. The computation of focal length for the experimental setup can be written as

$$f = \frac{(V_i - V_{i0})z_c}{x_c} = \frac{66.67 \times 50}{8} = 416.7 \text{ (pixels)} \tag{2.17}$$

where x_c is the measure of the center-to-center distance between the adjacent squares in the calibration chart using the world coordinate unit.

Calibration Parameters

The depth information can be obtained by using the computed focal length and Equation 2.2. Images of calibration markers were recorded at various distances from the endoscope (40, 60, 70, 80, and 90 mm). (Extensions of this experiment for tracking surgical tools are presented in Chapter 3.) The experiment data are shown in Table 2.3. The error is within 3 mm, fulfilling laparoscopic surgery application requirements quite well.

TABLE 2.3 Experimental Results Showing Comparison of Computed Distance of Endoscope to the Calibration Marker with the Actual Distance at Various Locations

No.	Actual Distance (mm)	Calculated Distance (mm)	Errors (mm)
1	40	42.5	2.5
2	60	60.5	0.5
3	70	69.4	0.6
4	80	78.1	1.9
5	90	88.2	1.8

TABLE 2.4 Variation in Least-Square Total Error with Respect to the Order of Expansion Polynomial

Polynomial Order *n*	**1**	**3**	**5**	**7**
Least squares total error	1.9909	0.1445	0.04196	0.04113

Distortion Correction

In order to experimentally demonstrate the result of the proposed distortion correction procedure, the same calibration chart containing a rectangular array of black squares was utilized.

The testing chart was placed perpendicularly to the optical axis 40 mm away from the tip of the endoscope. The left image in Figure 2.10 shows the captured image. We compute the polynomial coefficients using the method proposed previously, and the corrected image is shown in Figure 2.10(a). It can be seen that the image is magnified after correction and the lines are straightened, especially in the peripheral part.

The least squares total error reduces when the order of the polynomial becomes higher. It was found that the variation in least-square total error was negligible beyond the third polynomial order (see Table 2.4). Although distortion correction is performed once at the beginning of surgery, the third polynomial order was selected, which offers a balance between computation time and error.

The relationship between the radial distance of the testing points from the real image center before and after distortion correction is shown in Table 2.5. In the experiment, squares lying along the same row are selected. As shown in Figure 2.11, squares lying along the long black line in the same row are selected.

TABLE 2.5 Radial Distance of Testing Points from the Real Image Center before and after Distortion Correction

Actual Radial Distance (pixels)	**22**	**56**	**84**	**112**	**140**
Radial distance (pixels) (before correction)	22	55	82	108	134
Radial distance (pixels) (after correction)	22.4009 (22)	56.0093 (56)	84.0326 (84)	111.6783 (112)	140.1538 (140)

SUMMARY

In this chapter, some of the surgical tools used in performing conventional MIS were introduced. Specifically, some of the most common surgical components present in any conventional MIS theater are the endoscope, camera, and viewing monitor. These tools were further studied and analyzed as a part of the visual tracking system. Methods for obtaining various intrinsic parameters of the endoscope such as its focal length and optical scale factor were presented. In addition, methods for obtaining an undistorted image through the endoscope were presented, which can offer a uniform and consistent metric association to various locations on the endoscopic images. The methods in this chapter were also experimentally validated in order to demonstrate their practical implications.

CHAPTER 3

Marker-Based Tracking

THIS CHAPTER PRESENTS THE visual tracking method that uses a specific design of marker located on the surgical tool. Using the intrinsic and calibrated parameters of the endoscope, it is shown how the position of the surgical tool in the field of view of the endoscope can be interpreted as the spatial information of its marker. This information can be used to monitor the movements of the surgical tools used both by surgeons and resident trainees during surgical operations or various training phases. This chapter also shows how 2-D tracking information of the surgical tool can be used as an approach for the surgeon to interact with the overlay menu to access medical information about the patient. The next chapter will show extensions on how 3-D tracking of the tool can be used as part of image-guided surgery, where the surgeon can manipulate overlaid 3-D graphical objects containing medical information on the surgical site. This chapter also presents the gesture recognition approach, where, using the shape of the surgical tool tip as a natural marker, various gestures of the tool can be used as part of the surgeon–computer interface (SCI).

DESIGN OF MARKER

There exist many types of tracking methods, such as *optical flow* (2-D distribution of apparent velocities that can be associated with the variation of brightness patterns on the image), *feature points* correspondence, and *model-based tracking* (see Chapter 1). Due to the diversity in the designs of surgical tools, it is usually more challenging to locate them using shape analysis. To address this problem, in this chapter, a black strip marker is designed. The marker is attached to the tip of the instrument and then identified during the tracking task.

In general, the tracking task includes recognition of markers and computation of their relative position in the camera coordinate frame.

In real surgery, the surgical instrument may enter the field of view of the endoscope from various incision points with different positions and different angles. As stated, utilization of shape analysis and pattern matching would be infeasible since no stationary, static reference shape can be defined during the dynamic movements of the surgical tool. Instead, information regarding image contrast is used for segmenting artificial markers in order to determine their position in the surgical field of view. Two factors should be considered in the design of a marker. For one thing, in real-time image tracking, the marker should not be too complex and should be easily located in the field of view. In addition, due to the restriction on the size of the surgical instruments, the size of the marker should be chosen accordingly. Considering these constrains, there exist a number of possible design options. For example, one possible design could be the attachment of several circular markers to the tips of the instruments (Funda et al. 1996). However, utilization of this design is limited to 2-D computation of the positional information and lacks the framework for computing the spatial information associated with the surgical tool tip.

Figure 3.1 shows a marker design consisting of strips that can be used for obtaining the 3-D positional information of the surgical tool tip. The strips are of the same size, with the width *d*, and are attached to a tool with the diameter *M*. Points *P1*, *P2*, and *P3* are the centers of each strip projected onto the image plane.

A marker design with the configuration of Figure 3.1 has several advantages. First, the shape of the marker is simple, and it can offer a high contrast with the instruments and the surgical background, which can

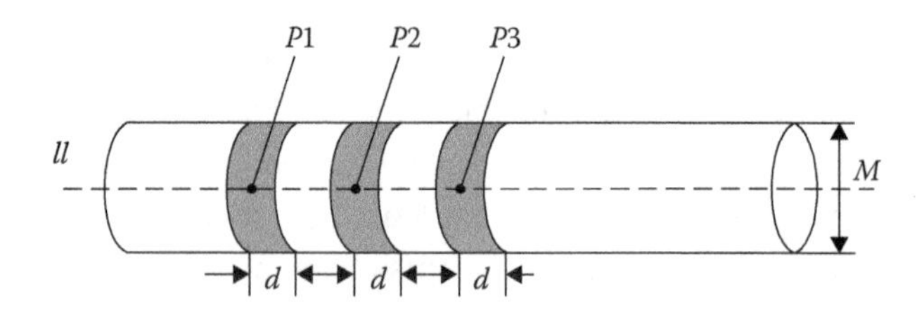

FIGURE 3.1 Proposed design of a marker consisting of a number of strips.

facilitate its visual segmentation for further analysis. Second, to acquire the depth information, the diameter of the tool can be used as a key identifier that can be used in the computational process. That is, regardless of the rotation of the surgical tool about its axis (*ll* in Figure 3.1), this parameter will remain unchanged in the endoscopic images. Finally, even with occlusion by organs or other instruments (i.e., when there is no visual information about one or two, or more, of these strips), it is still possible to acquire positional information from the remaining strips. However, the strip size cannot be designed too narrow or too small, otherwise it will make it difficult to locate the marker.

During the tracking procedure, one of the points among *P1*, *P2*, or *P3* can be located that is not being occluded and is the closest one to the tip of the surgical tool. In order to determine which strip is the closest one to the tip, we can compare their diameter M value in the image (see Figure 3.1). Generally, the smallest M is the one closest to the surgical site. Because of the perspective property under the endoscopic view (objects closer to the endoscope will appear bigger than same-size objects located farther away), generally, a rectangular strip marker appears as the shape shown in Figure 3.2a (a closed trapezoid shape *ABCD*). The length between A and B is selected to represent the diameter of the surgical tool (see Figure 3.2b), and point E as the blob center is one of the tracking points. Based on the changes of point E in directions V_i and V_j in the image plane and the calibration parameters described in Chapter 2, the real world can be computed. Using changes of the tool diameter length M in the image plane, the relative distance between the endoscope and the marker located on the surgical tool can be obtained.

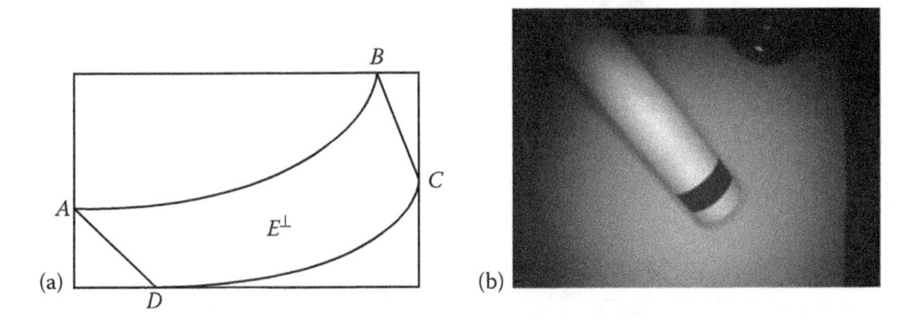

FIGURE 3.2 (a) The notion of using blob analysis for locating the desired points in the projected image of the marker; (b) the actual image of an endoscopic marker.

UNIT CONVERSION

The results presented in Chapter 2 can be used to estimate the z coordinate of the marker in millimeters; however, the measured x and y coordinates are computed in pixels. In order for the measured units to match, the unit has to be converted (with a conversion factor) from pixels in the frame buffer to physical units. The conversion factor represents the number of millimeters per pixel, and it is a function of the z coordinate (depth) of the surgical tool. For example, when the surgical tool is close to the laparoscope, it takes a larger number of pixels to represent the position of the marker. In comparison, the marker can be represented with fewer pixels when the surgical tool is farther away from the endoscope. In other words, the number of pixels representing 1 mm varies with the z coordinate representing the position of the surgical tool with respect to the endoscope. As a result, the z coordinate of the positional marker needs to be determined first in order to associate a correct conversion factor for mapping the x and y coordinates from pixel units to millimeters.

Pixel-to-Millimeter Conversion

To determine the pixel-to-millimeter conversion factor at various depth distances, a marker with a pair of black circles is placed under the endoscopic camera system at 18 different distances (Figure 3.3). The *in vitro* experiment is carried out so that the actual physical distance can also be measured using a physical instrument. The centers of the two black circles on the marker are separated by 10 mm. At each of the 18 different

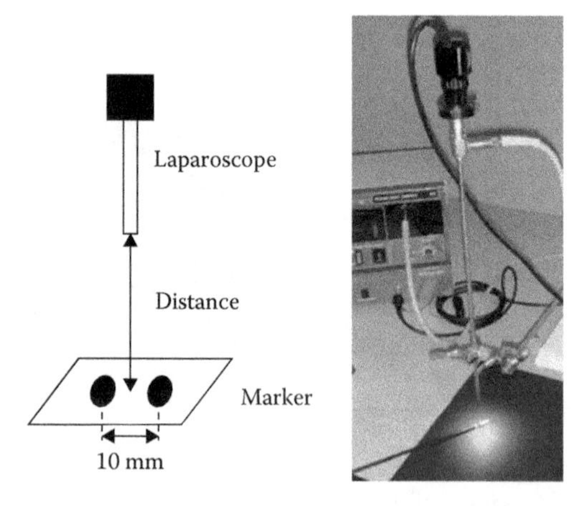

FIGURE 3.3 Setup for determining the pixel-to-millimeter conversion factor at various distances.

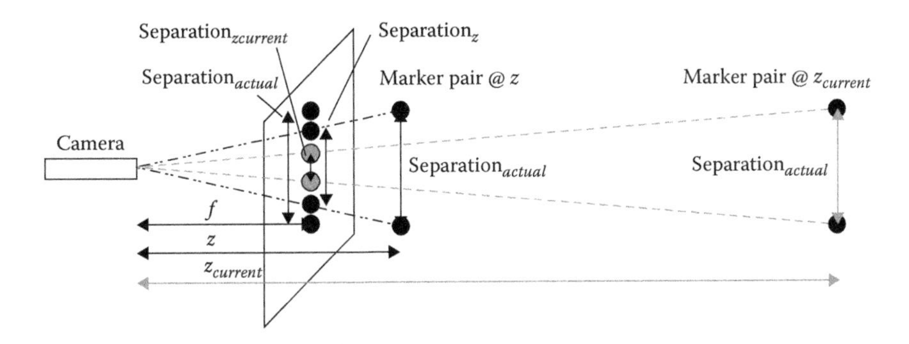

FIGURE 3.4 Relationship between separation, distance z, and focal length/plane.

distances, the 10 mm separation between the centers of the black circles would be shown to be different. The number of pixels representing the 10 mm separation is recorded for each of the distances.

Figure 3.4 shows a pinhole camera model of the experimental setup. The focal length f is the distance between the image plane and the camera. Assuming the marker with the pair of dots is parallel to the image plane, the further away the marker is to the camera, the smaller the separation appears on the screen, and vice versa. This is illustrated by separation$_{zcurrent}$ and separation$_z$, where separation$_{zcurrent}$ is the separation that appears on the screen when the marker is placed at $z_{current}$, and separation$_z$ is the separation that appears on the screen when the marker is placed at z. When the marker is placed at a distance of $z = 41$ mm, separation$_z$ appears as 100 pixels on the screen. Consequently, the conversion factor can be computed to be 1 mm:10 pixels. When the marker is placed at $z_{current} = 100$ mm, the separation$_{zcurrent}$ appears as 35 pixels on the screen. The resulting conversion factor is 1 mm:3.5 pixels, which is much larger than that at $z = 41$ mm.

The numbers of pixels appearing on screen that represent the 10 mm actual separation at different distances between 30 and 200 mm are recorded. In general, the number of pixels reduces by 50% as distance doubles, which is supported by the recorded experimental data. The overall inverse-proportional relationship between separation and distance from the collected data is shown in Figure 3.5.

To convert the estimated x and y coordinates from pixels to millimeters, the appropriate pixel-to-millimeter conversion factor can be retrieved from Figure 3.5 as a function of the z coordinate estimate of the surgical tool. The x_{pixel} and y_{pixel} coordinates, estimated by blob analysis in pixels, are converted to x_{mm} and y_{mm} in millimeters as follows:

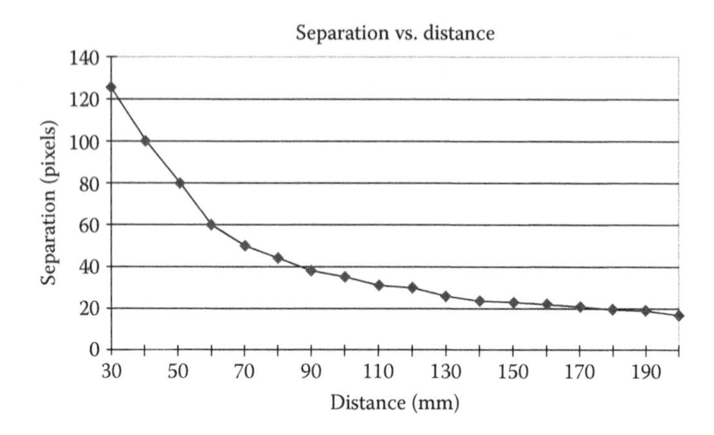

FIGURE 3.5 Number of pixels appearing on screen representing 10 mm actual separation versus distance.

$$x_{\text{mm}} = \left(x_{\text{pixel}} - x_{\text{offset}}\right) \times \text{conversion factor} \tag{3.1}$$

$$y_{\text{mm}} = \left(y_{\text{pixel}} - y_{\text{offset}}\right) \times \text{conversion factor} \tag{3.2}$$

where x_{offset} and y_{offset} are offsets between the screen frame and camera frame in pixels. The origin of the screen frame is in the top-left corner of the image window, while the origin of the camera frame is directly below the camera at the center of the image, hence the offsets. Where an estimated z coordinate does not match one of the recorded distances, a linear interpolation is utilized. For example, if the estimated z coordinate is 74 mm, which is between 70 mm and 80 mm, then the approximate screen separation is

$$50 + (40 - 50) \times \left(\frac{74 - 70}{80 - 70}\right) = 50 + (-10) \times 0.4 = 46 \text{ pixels}$$

Consequently, the conversion factor is 1 mm:4.6 pixels.

Results and Analysis

In vitro analysis of the proposed unit conversion is carried out in the environment with 10×10 mm grids on a piece of black paper as the background (Figure 3.3b). The surgical grasper is placed on the background paper such that its attached marker can be located directly on top of one of the grids.

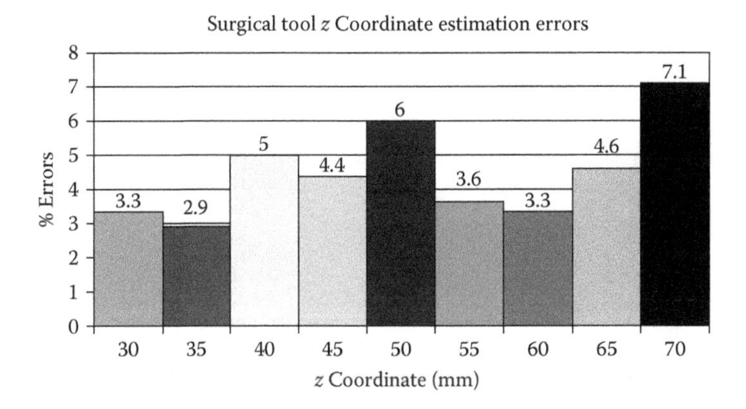

FIGURE 3.6 Estimation of distance of the surgical tool tip with respect to the endoscope reference frame with the associated estimation error.

Although the conversion factor table works for surgical tool distances from 30 to 200 mm, the range for the experimental evaluation is selected to be between 30 and 70 mm. With the brightness of the light source set at 35 lx, the light becomes too dim at distances beyond 70 mm, which makes the position marker too dim for it to be recognized. For simplicity, lens distortion is also ignored in our experimental studies of this section.

The surgical tool is placed at a distance between 30 and 70 mm below the laparoscope. Figure 3.6 shows the estimate of the z coordinate. The smallest error is 2.9% at 35 mm, and the largest error is 7.1% at 70 mm. The average error is only 4.5%, which falls within the range of acceptable performance.

To estimate the error in an automated localization and tracking of the surgical tool using the proposed method, several other measurement techniques were also utilized in order to verify its overall performance. Beside direct measurement (using a ruler), a 3-D electromagnetic tracking system (Ascension 2016; a position and orientation measurement system) was also used to measure positional data.

Four points with different locations were selected in the field of view of the endoscope. One of the strips of the surgical tool was manually placed at these locations. Since we are using the diameter of the surgical tool for computing the depth information, the 3-D marker information extraction method is applied to various surgical tool orientations in the endoscopic field of view. For the experiment, we captured 10 frames in every location. The mean tracking error is defined as the average difference over a whole sequence between the actual measured location and the positional

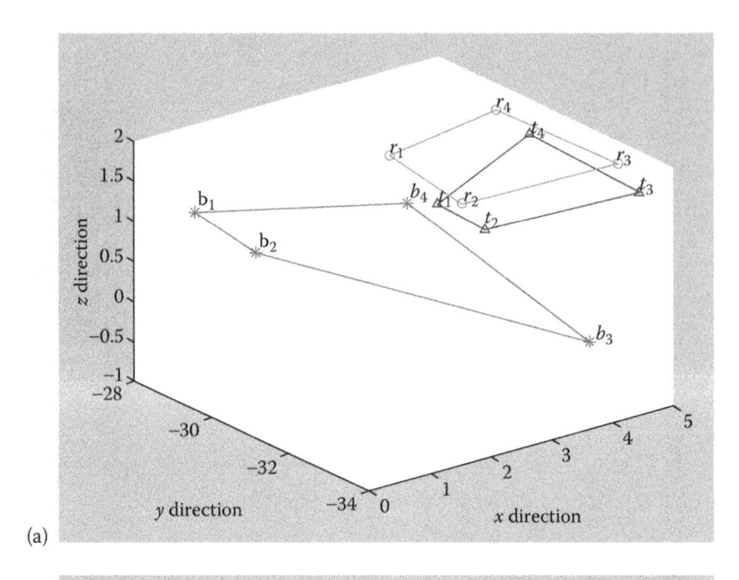

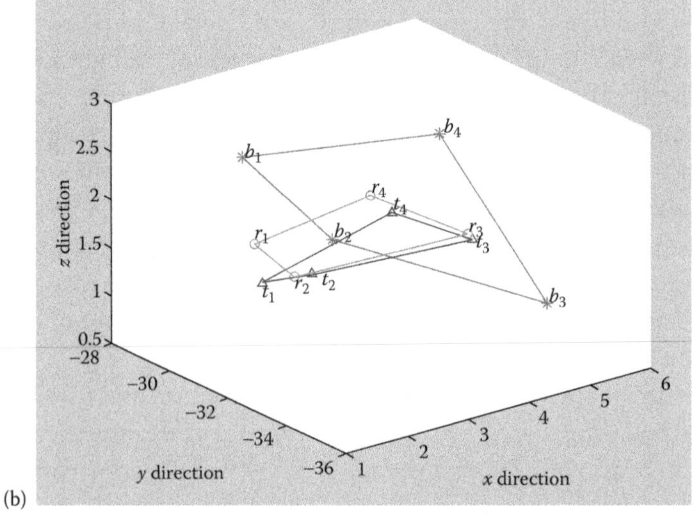

FIGURE 3.7 Comparison of tracking results (initial b represents external 3-D sensor, t represents the results of visual tracker and r represents the actual position measures). (a) The results of the surgical tool entering the endoscopic field of view at 0°; (b) when the tool enters the field at 45°.

information obtained from the proposed tracking method. A similar approach is applied for measuring tool positional information using a 3-D electromagnetic tracking system. The results of this experimental comparison are shown in Figure 3.7 and Table 3.1. The error is measured in centimeters and in the x, y, and z directions (in the World coordinate units).

TABLE 3.1 Average Error in Marker-Based Tracking of Surgical Tools

	Mean Tracking Error (cm)					
	x Direction		*y* Direction		*z* Direction	
Sequence No. (10 Frames)	**3-D Sensor**	**Image Tracking**	**3-D Sensor**	**Image Tracking**	**3-D Sensor**	**Image Tracking**
Point 1	−2.0817	−0.0286	1.7060	−1.2817	−0.6661	−0.2999
Point 2	−1.9400	−0.1123	2.2452	−0.7557	−0.7152	−0.1177
Point 3	−0.3100	−0.2132	0.2786	−0.8689	−2.2257	−0.1177
Point 4	−0.9635	0.0200	0.7644	−0.8301	−1.1250	−0.1177

From Figure 3.7, it can be seen that the image tracking results are better than employing an external measurement instrument such as a 3-D electromagnetic position and orientation measurement system. Part of the reason is the restriction that this measuring system can only be utilized in a nonmetallic environment. However, such restrictions cannot always be guaranteed in a conventional MIS operating room. In this experiment, the source of error for both of the tracking methods can also be related to the manual placement of the marker at the four calibration positions.

To account for the smaller field of view at shorter distances to the endoscope, the test points for the *x* and *y* coordinate estimations at distances 30 and 40 mm are chosen to be (10 mm, 10 mm), (−10 mm, 10 mm), (10 mm, −10 mm), and (−10 mm, −10 mm). Figure 3.8 shows an example of one of

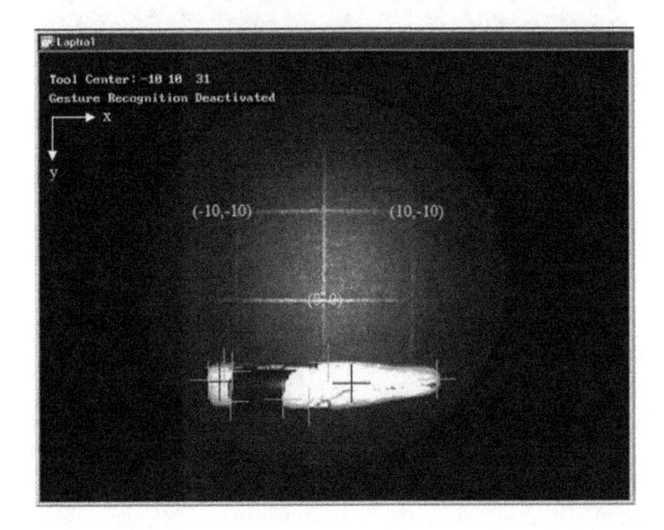

FIGURE 3.8 Experiment done at a distance of 30 mm to the endoscope with the marker placed at (−10, 10).

the tests done at a distance of 30 mm with illumination brightness set at 35 lx. The positional marker on the grasper is placed at (−10 mm, 10 mm). The converted *x* and *y* coordinates, which are the first two numbers of *Tool Center* shown in Figure 3.8, are recorded. The third number, 31 (shown on the top-left corner), is the estimated distance of the position marker. The black crosses mark the center of the positional marker and tool tip blobs. The gray crosses mark the four blob boundary points (*x_min*, *y_max_at_x_min*), (*x_max_at_y_max*, *y_max*), (*x_min_at_y_min*, *y_min*), and (*x_max*, *y_min_at_x_max*).

Test points (0 mm, 20 mm), (0 mm, −20 mm), (20 mm, 0 mm), and (−20 mm, 0 mm) are added for distances 50–70 mm due to the larger field of view. Figure 3.9 shows the wider field of view at a distance of 70 mm with the position marker at (0 mm, 0 mm). The complete *x* and *y* coordinates estimation test results are listed in Table 3.2. The first row shows

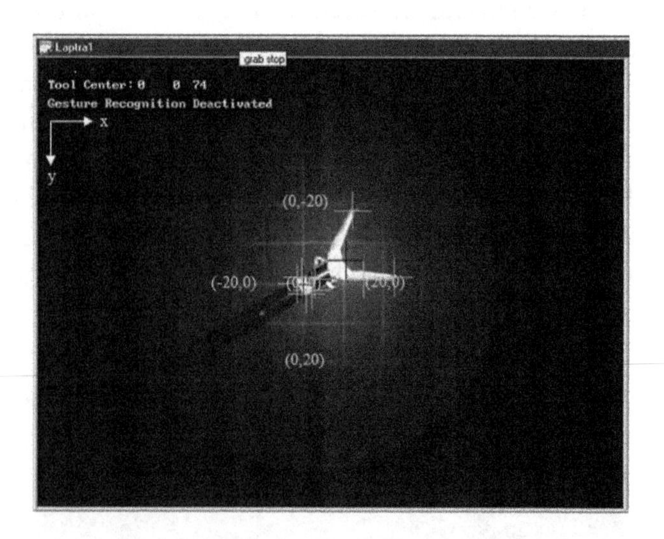

FIGURE 3.9 Wider field of view at a distance of 70 mm with the position marker at (0, 0).

TABLE 3.2 Test Results of Positional Markers (x, y) Coordinate Unit Conversion

	(*x*, *y*)							
Distance	**(10,10)**	**(−10,10)**	**(10,−10)**	**(−10,−10)**	**(0,20)**	**(0,−20)**	**(20,0)**	**(−20,0)**
30 mm	(9,11)	(−9,9)	(9,−8)	(−9,−9)				
40 mm	(10,9)	(−10,9)	(9,−9)	(−10,−11)				
50 mm	(9,9)	(−12,9)	(8,−11)	(−10,−10)	(0,19)	(1,−20)	(20,−1)	(−24,0)
60 mm	(12,9)	(−8,10)	(12,−10)	(−8,−10)	(1,18)	(0,−21)	(22,−1)	(−21,0)
70 mm	(13,8)	(−9,10)	(13,−10)	(−8,−10)	(−1,20)	(0,−20)	(22,0)	(−21,−1)

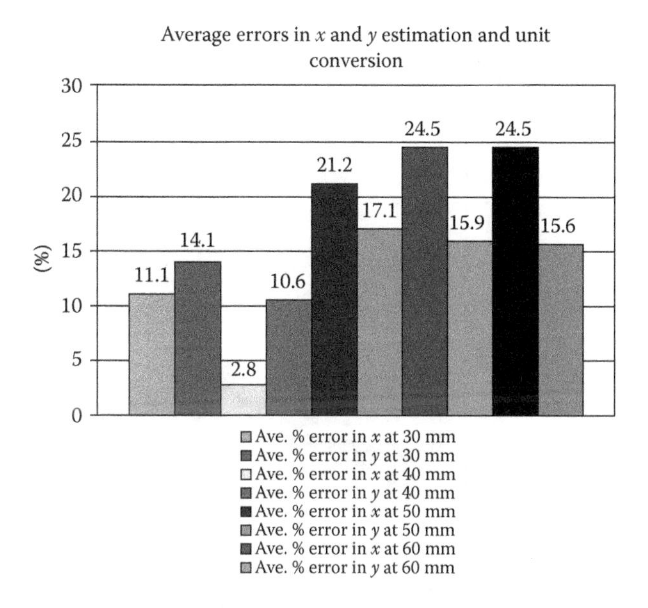

FIGURE 3.10 Average errors in coordinate estimation and unit conversion at each distance.

the test points, and the first column shows the different distances. The surgical grasper is placed on the grid such that the center of the positional marker sits right on top of the test points.

The tests show the overall average x and y coordinate estimation and unit conversion errors are 19.3% and 15.2% for x and y, respectively. The average errors in x and y at each distance are shown in Figure 3.10. For example, the first two bars from the left show that, for x and y at 30 mm, the average coordinate estimation and unit conversion errors are 11.1% and 14.1%. Recall from earlier results that the choice of conversion factor depends on the estimated z coordinate; therefore, the x and y coordinate estimation and unit conversion errors contain inherited errors from the z coordinate estimation.

GESTURE RECOGNITION OF SURGICAL TOOLS

One of the applications of the notion of marker-based tracking systems is gesture recognition. This application can provide the surgeon an interface with medical and visual information during the surgery. Shown in Figure 3.11 are nine commonly used surgical tools, including grasper, scissors, dissector, hook scissors, spoon forceps, claw forceps, needle holder, cauterizers, and fan retractors. All the surgical tools have an *open* state

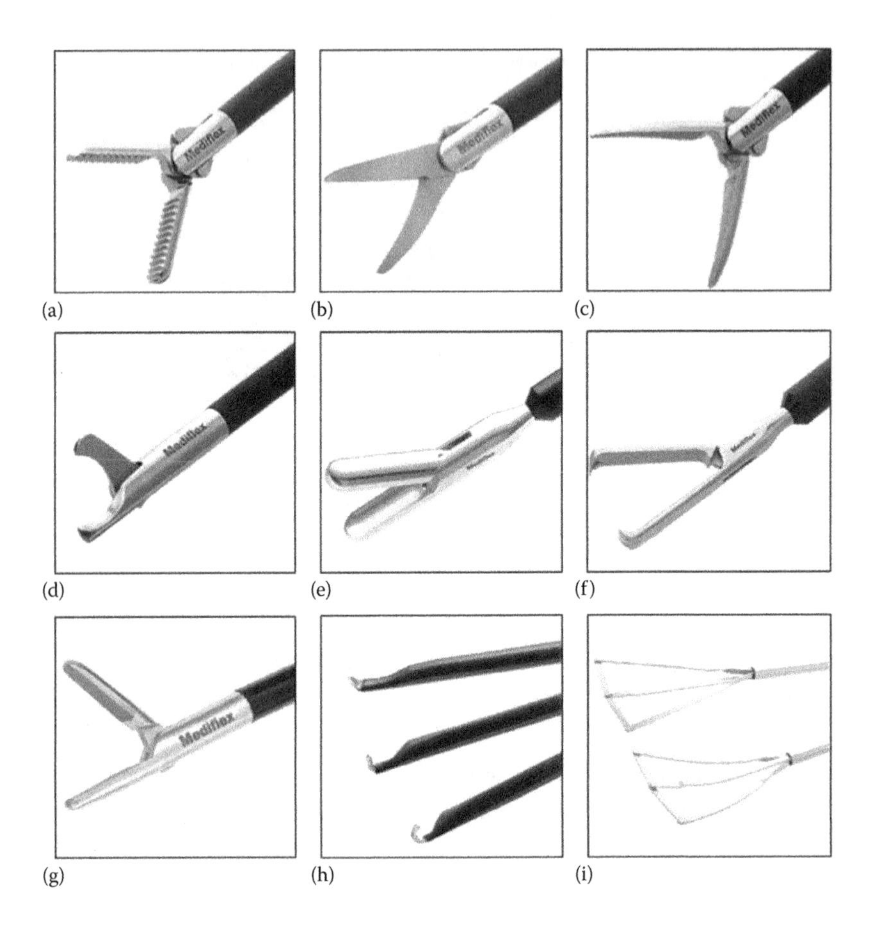

FIGURE 3.11 Nine commonly used surgical tools. (a) Grasper; (b) scissors; (c) dissector; (d) hook scissors; (e) spoon forceps; (f) claw forceps; (g) needle holder; (h) cauterizers; (i) fan retractors.

and a *closed* state, except for the cauterizers and fan retractors. The multistate surgical tools can create more tool gestures than the cauterizers and fan retractors. In this study, we have chosen the surgical grasper and scissors, the two most commonly used multistate surgical instruments, for creating tool gestures. In addition to the open and closed states, multistate surgical tools can also have intermediate states such as *half-open*, *in the process of opening*, or *in the process of closing*. For simplicity, only the open and closed states are considered in our experiments.

Four single-tool gestures performed with either a grasper or a pair of scissors are shown in Figure 3.12a–d; four nonoverlapping double-tool gestures performed by combining grasper and scissors are shown in Figure 3.12e–h; and three overlapping double-tool gestures performed

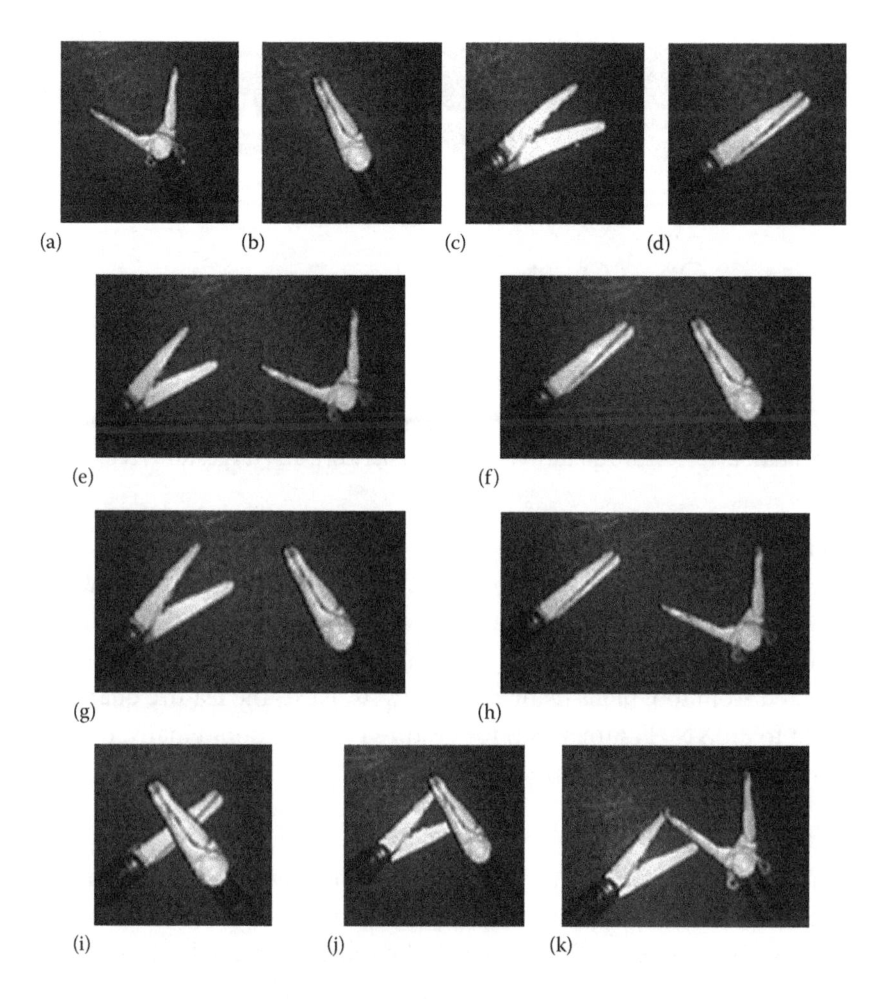

FIGURE 3.12 Various experimental gestures as a natural marker for surgical tool tips. (a) Open grasper; (b) closed grasper; (c) open scissors; (d) closed scissors; (e) both tools open; (f) both tools closed; (g) open scissors and closed grasper; (h) closed scissors and open grasper; (i) cross; (j) triangle; (k) double triangle.

with the combination of grasper and scissors are shown in Figure 3.12i–k (Hsu and Payandeh 2006; Hsu 2007).

The surgical tool gesture recognition function can be activated by manually pressing the activation switch on the handle of the surgical tool and terminated, for example, by performing a cross-tool gesture. The total sampling time of the function, which includes the time the surgical tools have to be held still and the time it takes for the system to recognize the tool gesture, can be considerably less than 1 s in the current state of computing hardware. Every acquired image, as shown in Figure 3.13, undergoes three

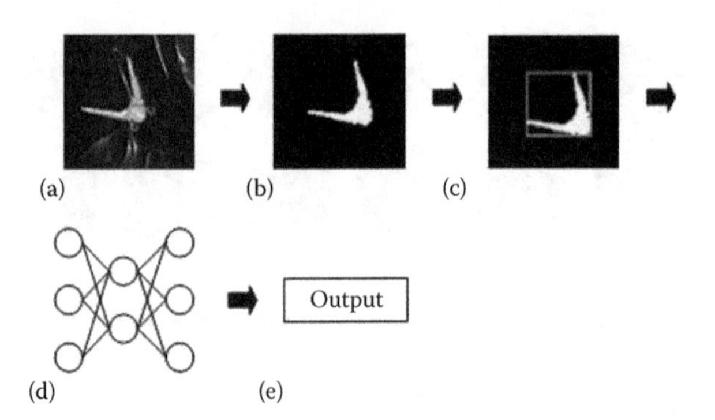

FIGURE 3.13 The surgical tool gesture method. (a) Input; (b) target tool segmentation; (c) feature quantity; (d) neural network and (e) gesture recognized.

different stages of processing, including tool segmentation, feature quantity extraction, and neural network (NN) gesture classification. In the first stage (Figure 3.13b), tool blobs are segmented with morphological filters and thresholding. In the second step (Figure 3.13c), feature quantities are extracted from tool blobs using blob analysis. Next, the feature quantities are fed to an NN (Figure 3.13d) for gesture classification. Finally, the surgical tool gesture is recognized, as shown in Figure 3.13e.

Target Tool Segmentation

Segmentation refers to the process of extracting meaningful regions from images. Such regions typically correspond to objects of interest or to their parts. Numerous researchers have studied and developed segmentation methods in order to reduce the undesirable effects of background information and to retain the objects of interest in images. One of the most popular approaches to target segmentation is the thresholding method (Sahoo et al. 1988). In simple implementations, segmentation is determined by a single parameter known as the *intensity threshold*. In a single pass, each pixel in the image is compared with this threshold. If the intensity of the pixel is higher than the threshold, the pixel is set to white in the output. If it is lower than the threshold, it is set to black.

Contour-based algorithms are also commonly used in segmentation. Contour-based segmentation methods use edge or boundary information to detect features of interest in an image. Kass et al. (1988) proposed the *snakes* model based on the deformation of an initial contour or surface toward the boundary of the object to be detected. The minima of the deformation energy function are obtained at the boundary of the object.

Color can also be used to segment objects from the background. Tai and Song (2004) apply a histogram method for background removal before segmenting moving vehicles in a vision-based traffic monitoring system via thresholding. Using statistical tools, the background image can be constructed from the histogram of individual pixels in an image sequence. It is assumed that, in a grayscale image, the pixel intensity that is most frequently recorded within a certain intensity range in the image sequence is the intensity of the background pixel. Removing the pixels with that certain intensity would remove the background.

Mathematical morphology is also a tool for extracting image components that are useful in the representation and description of a region's shape, such as boundaries, skeletons, and the convex hull (Gonzalez and Wood 2002). The framework of mathematical morphology is based on set theory. As such, morphology offers a unified and powerful approach to numerous image-processing problems, including object segmentation. Xuan et al. (1998) employ a two-step scheme for automatic object detection in computed radiography (CR) images utilizing morphological filters to extract the foreign objects and active contour models to outline the foreign objects. First, various structuring elements of the morphological filters are applied to effectively distinguish the foreign object candidates from the complex background structures. Second, active contour models are employed to accurately outline the morphological shapes of suspicious foreign objects such as tumors to further reduce the rate of false alarms.

Mathematical morphology is a geometrical approach to signal processing that can easily deal with shape, size, contrast, and connectivity (Salembier and Pardas 1994). Moreover, morphological operations can be efficiently implemented in both software and hardware environments. This point is of prime importance because the major bottleneck in segmentation is the complexity and computational load of the segmentation step. In other words, the simple and efficient nature of mathematical morphology can keep the processing time short, which is important in the time-critical surgery environment. With efficiency and processing time in mind, in this section thresholding and mathematical morphology are our selected methods for target tool tip segmentation. The performance of simple thresholding and morphology with thresholding are compared at the end of this chapter.

The first stage of the target tool segmentation method in our experiment is thresholding. Every pixel in the grayscale input image (Figure 3.13a) is compared with a fixed threshold value. Pixels with intensity values higher

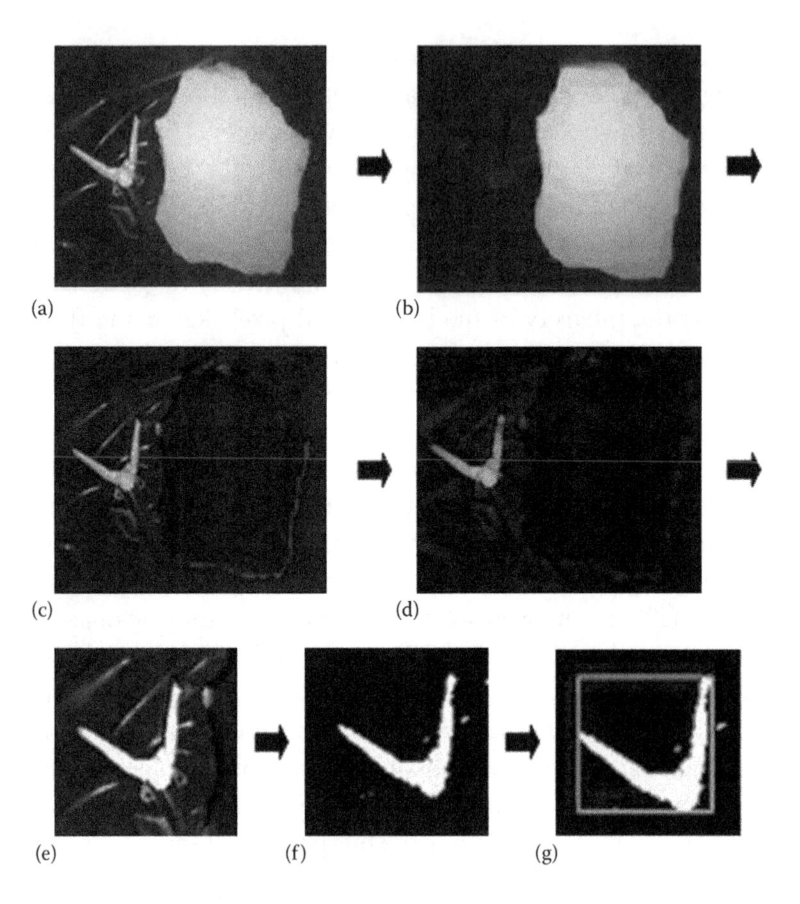

FIGURE 3.14 Target tool segmentation with morphological operations and thresholding. (a) Input image A; (b) $A \circ B_1$; (c) $A = A - (A \circ B_1)$; (d) $A \circ B_2$; (e) $A + (A \circ B_2)$; (f) thresholding; (g) target tool segmented.

than the threshold value are set to white, and pixels with intensity values lower than the threshold value are set to black. The threshold value is chosen based on preliminary testing results with the brightness of the light source set to 35 lx. The output is a binary image with the target tool segmented, as shown in Figure 3.13b.

The second method, the mathematical morphology method with thresholding, takes the same grayscale input image, and suppresses the background while retaining the size and location information of the target tool with morphological filters. The image then goes through thresholding, leaving only the target tool in the binary output image, as shown in Figure 3.13b. The morphological operation used in this method is the background reduction described by Xuan et al. (1998), which removes background objects larger than the target tool, and a modified background reduction, which removes background objects smaller than the target tool. Background reduction is defined as

$$\text{Background reduction} = A - (A \circ B_1) \tag{3.3}$$

where:

- A is the input image shown in Figure 3.13a
- B_1 is a square structuring element whose size is larger than the target tool of any shape
- $\circ$ is the grayscale opening operation, which is defined as

$$A \circ B = (A \ominus B) \oplus B \tag{3.4}$$

where $\oplus$ and $\ominus$ are grayscale dilation and erosion operations (Appendix II).

Figure 3.14a is the grayscale input image that contains the target tool, some small bright spots in the background, and a large piece of white paper. The result of the first step of background reduction, $A \circ B_1$, is shown in Figure 3.14b, where the target tool and small white spots are removed, and only the large piece of white paper remains. Then the complete result of background reduction is shown in Figure 3.14c, which is the difference between Figure 3.14a and Figure 3.14b. In Figure 3.14c, the large piece of white paper has been removed, leaving only the target tool and small bright spots.

To remove the background noise shown in Figure 3.14c, we changed the subtraction in Equation 3.3 to addition to form a modified background reduction as follows:

$$\text{Modified background reduction} = A + (A \circ B_2) \tag{3.5}$$

where A is now the image of Figure 3.14c, and B_2 is a square structuring element that is smaller than the target tool.

$A \circ B_2$ produces a grayscale image of the target tool, as shown in Figure 3.14d, where all the background white spots are removed and only the target tool is left. Then, instead of subtracting Figure 3.14d from image Figure 3.14c as in background reduction, Figure 3.14d is added to Figure 3.14c, as in Equation 3.5. The result is Figure 3.14e, with almost all pixels of the target tool saturated; that is, the intensity values of the pixels are at 255. In other words, the target tool is purely white, which makes it stand out among all other objects in the image.

The grayscale image is then converted to a binary image by thresholding. Since the intensity values for almost all the target tool pixels are at the maximum 255 after the modified background reduction, the threshold value can be set close to the maximum. The higher threshold value will eliminate all the small background bright spots, leaving only the target tool in the image, as shown in Figure 3.14f. This completes the target tool segmentation stage, and binary image Figure 3.14g is ready for the feature quantities extraction stage.

In summary, the input grayscale image first undergoes background reduction to remove background objects larger than the target tool. To eliminate background objects smaller than the target tool, modified background reduction is applied to the image. The resulting intensity values of the target tool pixels are at the maximum 255, which allows the threshold value to be set high to eliminate the leftover smaller background objects. Finally, the target tool is segmented, and the binarized output image only contains the target tool blob ready for the feature quantities extraction stage. At this stage, the threshold value, lighting conditions, surgical tool orientations, and background tissue reflections can all affect how well the shape of the segmented target tool is preserved. Less well-preserved target tool blobs will result in less accurate feature quantities. Consequently, the tool gesture classification will be less accurate.

Feature Extraction

Feature quantities are quantitative representations of target tool blobs in the final binarized image of the target tool segmentation stage, shown in Figure 3.14g. They are distinctive informational qualities extracted from the target tool blobs that, together, allow the surgical tool gestures to be classified. Six feature quantities are defined and used in distinguishing the surgical tool gestures. The feature quantities form the input vector to the surgical tool gesture–classifying NN that is presented in the next section.

Four of the feature quantities that are defined and implemented are compactness, roughness, elongation, and Feret elongation. The fifth and sixth feature quantities are the maximum color change count and the minimum color change count. The maximum color change count is the maximum number of black-to-white and white-to-black color changes in the final binary image shown in Figure 3.14g. On the other hand, the minimum color change count is the minimum number of black-to-white and white-to-black color changes in the final binary image.

The definitions of the six feature quantities are as follows. *Compactness* is a measure of how close all particles in the blob are from one another. It is derived from perimeter and area. A circular blob is the most compact and is defined as having a compactness measure of 1.0 (the minimum); more convoluted shapes such as hexagons have higher values. For example, it was found that the open grasper shown in Figure 3.15a has a compactness of 4.5, which is higher than the 2.2 of the closed grasper shown in Figure 3.15b.

Roughness is a measure of the unevenness or irregularity of the surface of a blob. It is the ratio of the perimeter to the convex perimeter of a blob. Smooth convex blobs have a roughness of 1.0, whereas rough blobs have a higher value because their perimeter is bigger than their convex perimeter. For example, the roughness of the double triangle shown in Figure 3.16a is 1.6, which is higher than the 1.1 of the closed grasper shown in Figure 3.16b.

Elongation is equal to the ratio of the blob length to the blob breadth. These features are derived from area and perimeter, using the assumption that the blob area is equal to (length × breadth) and the perimeter is equal

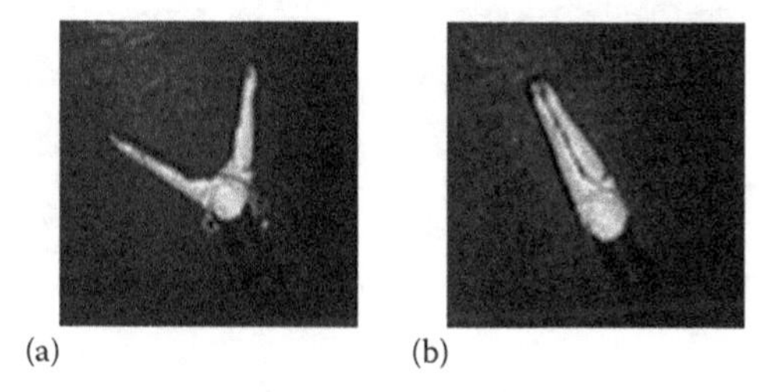

FIGURE 3.15 Compactness measure for the open and closed gestures of the surgical tool. (a) Open grasper compactness = 4.5; (b) closed grasper compactness = 2.2.

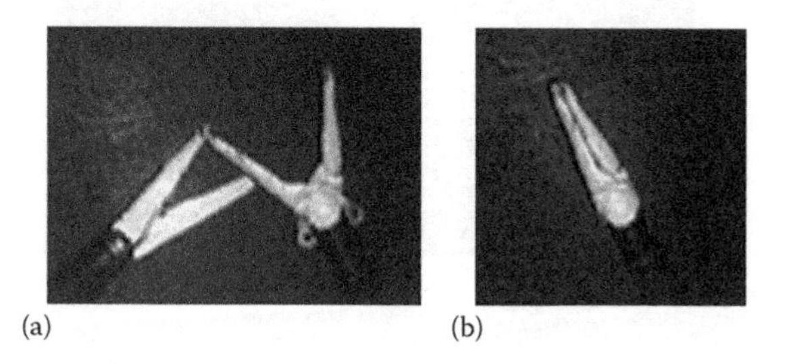

FIGURE 3.16 Roughness of the double triangle and closed grasper. (a) Double triangle roughness = 1.6; (b)closed grasper roughness = 1.1.

to (2[length + breadth]). Breadth is also known as width. This quantity is a better measurement for long and thin blobs. The open grasper shown in Figure 3.17a has an elongation of 11.8, while the closed grasper shown in Figure 3.17b has a much smaller elongation of 4.5. From the definition, the open grasper shown in Figure 3.17a should have a smaller elongation than the closed grasper in Figure 3.17b due to the larger breadth. The miscalculation may have resulted from the fact that the grasper tool tip blob is not as long and thin as the feature extraction function prefers. However, it was found that the miscalculation was consistent, suggesting that this feature quantity could still be used in classifying the tool gestures.

Feret elongation is equal to the ratio of the maximum Feret diameter to the minimum Feret diameter, which are determined by testing the diameter of the blob at several angles. This quantity is a better measurement for short and thick blobs. The open grasper shown in Figure 3.18a has a Feret elongation of 1.3, while the closed grasper shown in Figure 3.18b has a larger Feret elongation of 2.5.

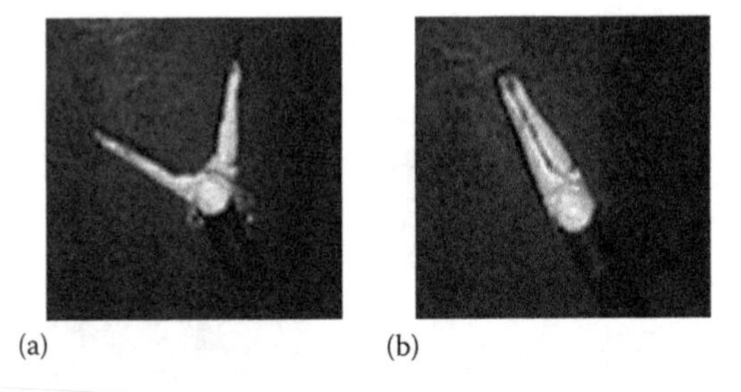

FIGURE 3.17 A measure of the elongation of an open grasper and a closed grasper. (a) Open grasper elongation = 11.8; (b) closed grasper elongation = 4.5.

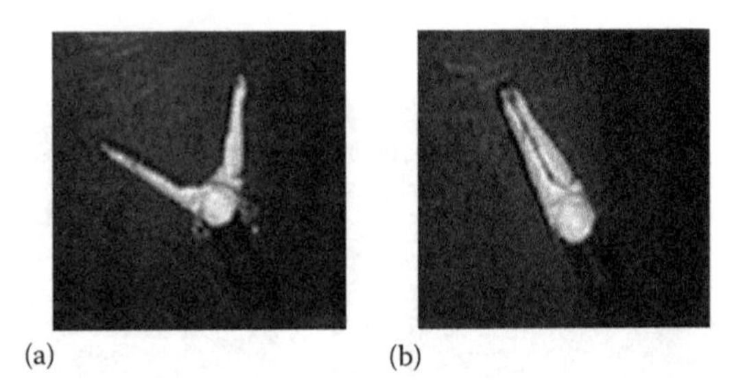

FIGURE 3.18 A measure of blob elongation using Feret elongation of an open grasper and a closed grasper. (a) Open grasper Feret elongation = 1.3; (b) close grasper Feret elongation = 2.5.

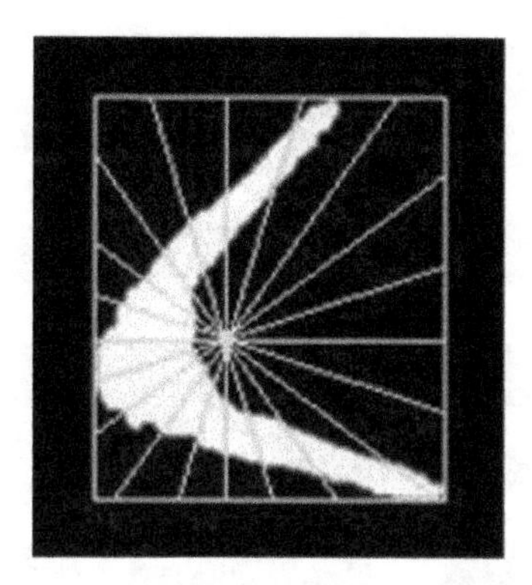

FIGURE 3.19 Ten scan lines drawn to determine the maximum and minimum color change counts in a surgical tool gesture.

Maximum and minimum color change counts are determined with the same function. The number of white-to-black or black-to-white color changes is counted along 10 scan lines, as shown in the binary image of an open grasper gesture in Figure 3.19. The center of the scan is where the 10 scan lines intersect, which is also the blob center determined by blob analysis.

Surgical tools can enter the field of view of the endoscope at various angles. Although performing a 360° scan would guarantee finding the maximum and minimum number of color changes, it would cost extra processing time. To minimize the processing overhead, the minimum number of scan lines is decided based on the analysis that is depicted in Figure 3.20.

Figure 3.20a shows an open grasper gesture. The two yellow lines intersecting at the blob center divide the plane into four regions. Any scan line drawn from the region labeled 2 that intersects the blob center will encounter two black-to-white or white-to black color changes. Similarly, any scan line drawn from the region labeled 4 that intersects the blob center would encounter four black-to-white or white-to black color changes. In the open grasper case, the low color change count is two, and the high color change count is four. The two yellow lines are almost perpendicular to each other. To accurately count the maximum and minimum number of color changes regardless of the yaw angle of the surgical tool, the angles between each scan line have to be smaller than 90°. Consequently, drawing three scan lines 60° to each other would guarantee finding the maximum and minimum number of color changes.

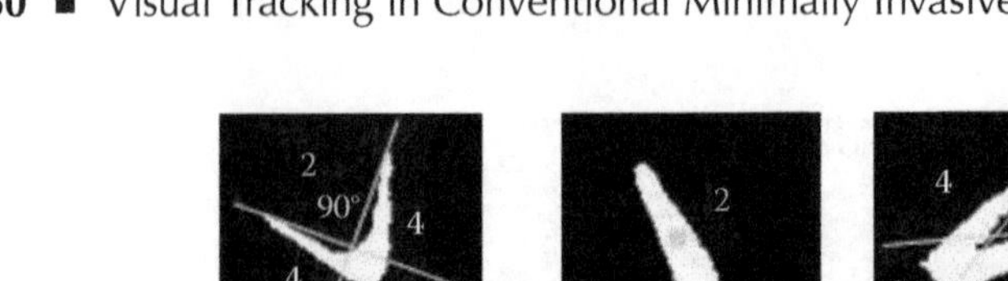

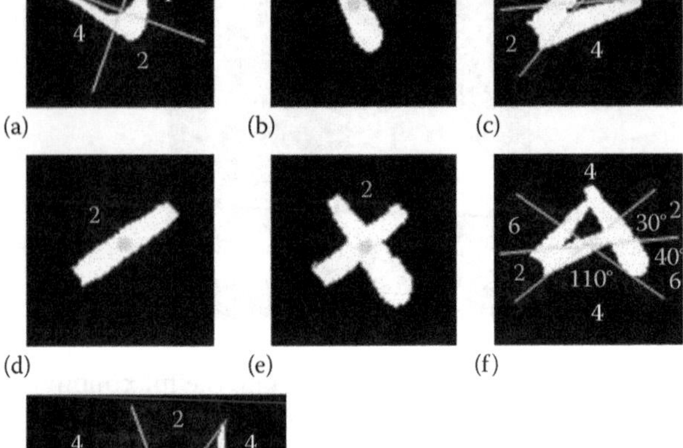

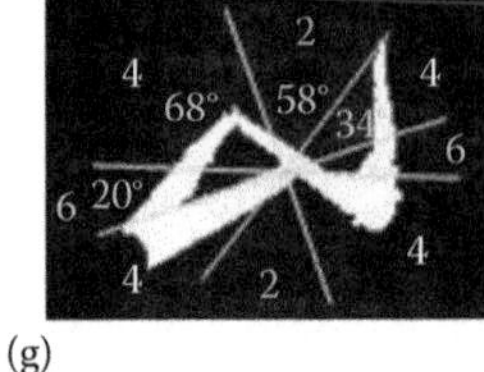

FIGURE 3.20 Color change count regions for the single-tool gestures and the overlapping double-tool gestures. (a) Open grasper; (b) closed grasper; (c) open scissors; (d) closed scissors; (e)cross; (f) triangle; (g) double triangle.

Both of the maximum color change count and minimum color change count for the closed grasper gesture in Figure 3.20b, the closed scissors gesture in Figure 3.20d, and the cross gesture in Figure 3.20e are two. As long as the scan line intersects the blob center, the color change count is always two regardless of the angle. As a result, only one scan line is needed for these three cases.

The open scissors gesture shown in Figure 3.20c is similar to the open grasper case, except the angle between the two dividing lines is about 45°. Thus, it would require at least five scan lines 36° to each other to get the accurate maximum and minimum color change counts.

There are three possible color change counts—two, four, and six—for the triangle gesture shown in Figure 3.20f. To get the maximum color change count of six, the angles between the scan lines have to be smaller than 40°. Furthermore, to get the minimum color change count of two, the angles between the scan lines have to be smaller than 30°. Therefore, a minimum of seven scan lines 25.7° to each other is required.

The double triangle gesture shown in Figure 3.20g also has three possible color change counts. To get the minimum color change count of two, the angles between the scan lines have to be smaller than 58°. To get the maximum color change count of six, the angles between the scan lines have to be smaller than 20°. Therefore, a minimum of 10 scan lines 18° to each other is required.

The nonoverlapping double-tool gestures shown in Figure 3.12e–h are different combinations of the single-tool gestures in Figure 3.20a–d, so they are treated as two single-tool gestures. The minimum number of scan lines required for the nonoverlapping double-tool gestures, therefore, is the same as the single-tool gestures they consist of. To conclude, 10 is the minimum number of scan lines to determine the maximum and minimum color change counts in all 11 surgical tool gestures in the experiment.

The maximum and minimum color change counts effectively divide the surgical tool gestures into three groups. The first group consists of the open grasper and open scissors. Their maximum color change count is four, and their minimum color change count is two. The second group includes the closed grasper, closed scissors, and cross. Their maximum color change count and minimum color change count are both two. The third group consists of the triangle and double triangle. Their maximum color change count is six, and their minimum color change count is two. The surgical tool gesture classifier can use these two feature quantities to classify a given tool gesture into one of the three groups. It can then further classify the tool gesture based on the other four feature quantities.

However, finding the right number of maximum and minimum color changes is not always guaranteed. If the tool gesture is performed with the surgical tool making extreme roll, yaw, or pitch angles with respect to the coordinate frame located at the incision point, or if the shape of the target tool blob is not well preserved, the blob centers of the target tool blobs would be far away from the anticipated blob centers shown in Figure 3.20. As a result, the number of maximum and minimum color changes could be wrong. If the background is not completely removed, leaving small blobs around the target tool blob, the maximum and minimum number of color changes could also be wrong. Moreover, if the boundary of the target tool blob is not smooth, the maximum and minimum color change count could also be more than what they are supposed to be.

Gesture Pattern Recognition Using Artificial Neural Networks

At the center of a gesture pattern recognition system is the gesture classifier. There exist a number of approaches for pattern classification and learning (e.g., Nadler and Smith 1993; Bishop 2006). The gesture pattern classifier is responsible for interpreting the information gathered from the input gesture and classifying the gesture. An NN has the ability to make the best decision or approximation without understanding the complex underlying mechanism. Due to its parallel architecture, its fast response and computational times also make it very well suited to real-time systems (Bishop 2005).

NNs are made of units that can be described by single numbers—their *activation* values. Each unit generates an output signal based on its activation. Units are connected to each other very specifically, each connection having an individual *weight* (described by a scalar). Each unit sends its output value to all other units to which they have an outgoing connection. Through these connections, the output of one unit can influence the activations of other units. The unit receiving the connections calculates its activation by taking a *weighted sum* of the input signals (i.e., it multiplies each input signal with the weight that corresponds to that connection and adds these products). The output is determined by the activation function based on this activation (e.g., the unit generates output or *fires* if the activation is above a threshold value). Networks learn by changing the weights of the connections.

A feed-forward NN with one hidden layer is selected for gesture classification and recognition (FANN 2016; OpenNN 2016; Shimada et al. 2003; Kang et al. 2015). The proposed feed-forward NN has six neurons in the input layer, twenty neurons in the hidden layer, and seven neurons in the output layer. The input vector consists of the six feature quantities: compactness, roughness, elongation, Feret elongation, maximum color change count, and minimum color change count. The six feature quantities, which are six real numbers, are fed into the corresponding neurons in the input layer. The hidden layer neurons have sigmoid transfer functions. Twenty is determined to be the number of neurons that gives better results through testing. The output vector consists of the seven real numbers coming out of the seven neurons of the output layer. The seven numbers represent seven single-tool and overlapping double-tool gestures, including the open grasper, closed grasper, open scissors, and closed scissors shown in Figure 3.12a–d, and the cross, triangle, and double triangle shown in Figure 3.12i–k. The remaining four nonoverlapping double-tool gestures shown in Figure 3.12e–h are basically different combinations of the open and closed grasper and scissors. They are simply treated as two separate single-tool gestures, as shown in Figure 3.21, and they require the system to make two tool gesture recognition calls.

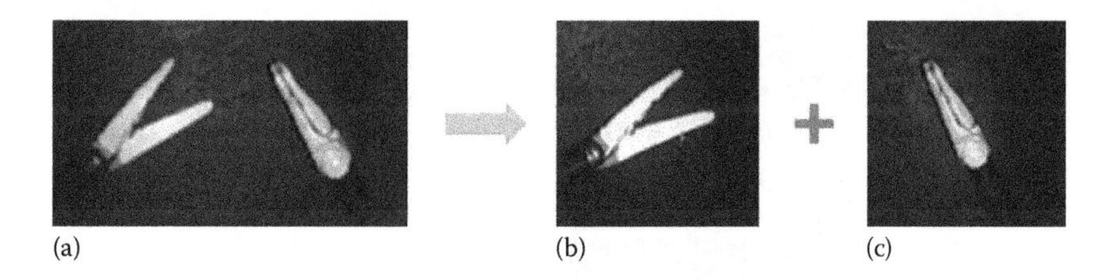

FIGURE 3.21 Nonoverlapping double-tool gesture: (a) *open scissors and closed grasper* being separated into two single-tool gestures: (b) *open scissors* and (c) *closed grasper.*

The NN is trained under supervised learning with backpropagation, in which the training data are fed into the network for many iterations, so that the network learns the relationship between the input and output. The goal is to determine a set of weights that minimizes the errors between the NN output and the training output. For the four single-tool gestures, there are seven sets of training data acquired from performing the tool gestures with different roll, pitch, and yaw angles. In the case of the *in vitro* study, we have adjusted the position of the endoscope, and the seven orientations represent the orientation angle of the endoscope at the point of entry, which emulates general cases of surgical tool surface orientation with respect to the image plane. Figure 3.22 shows the seven orientations: (a) natural position, (b) positive roll angle, (c) negative roll angle, (d) smaller negative pitch angle, (e) larger negative pitch angle, (f) positive yaw angle, and (g) negative yaw angle. The roll, pitch, and yaw angles of a surgical tool are defined with respect to a Cartesian coordinate frame located at the incision point of a surgical tool. Roll is a rotation about the axis of the surgical tool, while pitch and yaw are rotations about other axes perpendicular to the roll axis. For the three overlapping double-tool gestures, there are seven sets of training data acquired from performing the tool gestures at different positions. In Figure 3.23, the seven orientations are (a) middle, (b) up, (c) down, (d) left, (e) right, (f) near, and (g) far.

Each set of training data contains an input vector and an output vector. Each surgical tool gesture has seven sets of training data corresponding to the seven orientations. A total of 49 training data sets for the seven surgical tool gestures are used in training. An example training input vector for the open grasper gesture would be (4.34635, 1.2493, 11.568, 1.38424, 4.0, 2.0). The six numbers correspond to compactness, roughness, elongation, Feret elongation, maximum color change count, and minimum color change count. An example training output vector for the open gesture

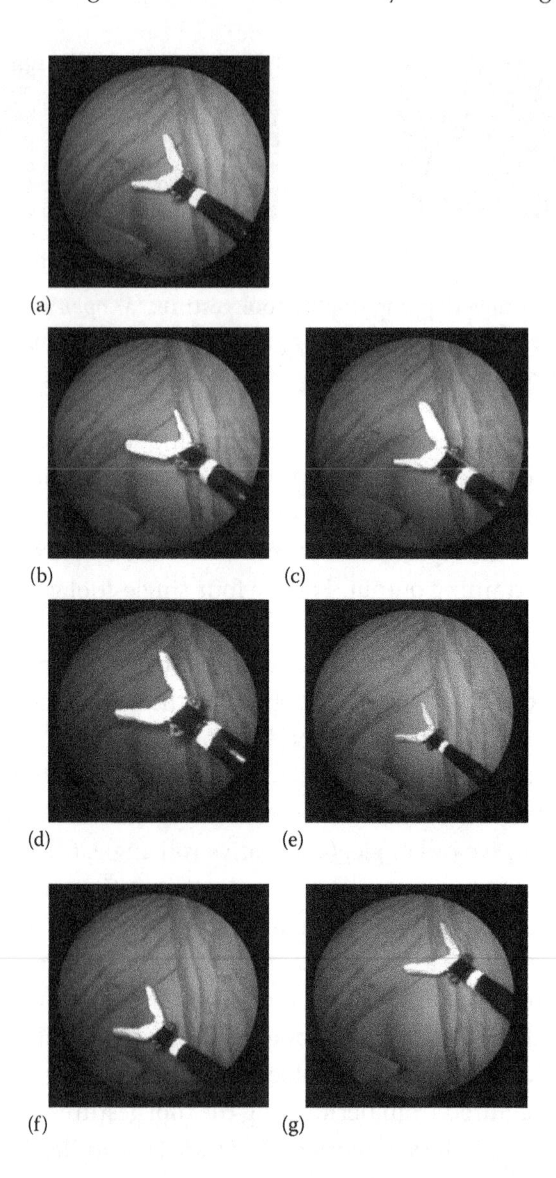

FIGURE 3.22 The seven orientations of single-tool gestures. (a) Natural position; (b) positive roll angle; (c) negative roll angle; (d) smaller negative pitch angle; (e) larger negative pitch angle; (f) positive yaw angle; (g) negative yaw angle.

would be (0.9, 0.1, 0.1, 0.1, 0.1, 0.1, 0.1). The seven numbers of the output vector represent open grasper, closed grasper, open scissors, closed scissors, cross, triangle, and double triangle. The first number, 0.9, which is significantly larger than the others, indicates that this is an open grasper gesture.

For each training iteration, one of the 49 training data sets is chosen. Then the input vector of the chosen training data set is fed to the NN. The errors between the output vector from the NN and the output vector of the chosen training data set are determined. The set of weights are then adjusted to minimize errors. In the preceding open grasper gesture example, the weights would be adjusted such that when the same training input vector is fed into the NN again, the first number in the NN output vector would be closer to 0.9, while the other six numbers would be closer to 0.1.

Results and Analysis

With the brightness of the light source set at 35 lx, the four single-tool gestures shown in Figure 3.12a–d are performed 10 times at each of the seven orientations and 10 times at ten different random orientations inside of the *in vitro* experimental setup (FLS 2016). The tool gestures are performed at distances between 30 and 70 mm, or the z coordinate as shown in Figure 3.3, in the field of view of the endoscope. As shown in Figure 3.22, the seven orientations include the natural position, positive roll angle, negative roll angle, smaller negative pitch angle, larger negative pitch angle, positive yaw angle, and negative yaw angle. The relative roll, pitch and yaw are defined with respect to a coordinate defined at the incision point. For example, roll rotation corresponds to the rotation of the surgical tool about its axis. A smaller negative pitch angle means the surgical tool is closer to the laparoscope. A larger pitch angle means the surgical tool is farther away from the laparoscope. In other words, the distance between the laparoscope and the surgical grasper is larger. The three overlapping double-tool gestures shown in Figure 3.12i–k are also performed 10 times at each of the seven orientations and 10 times at ten different random orientations inside the plastic stomach at distances between 30 and 70 mm. As shown in Figure 3.23, the seven orientations are middle, up, down, left, right, near, and far.

Figure 3.24 shows the open grasper gesture being recognized and the recognition rates for the seven orientations, all of which are 100%. The recognition rate for random orientations, which involves different combinations of various roll, pitch, and yaw angles, is 90%. Overall, the open grasper gesture can be recognized at a success rate of 98.75%. Being one of the basic single-tool gestures, the open grasper gesture is expected to have a high recognition rate.

Figure 3.25 shows the closed grasper gesture being recognized and the recognition rates for the natural, positive roll angle, negative roll angle,

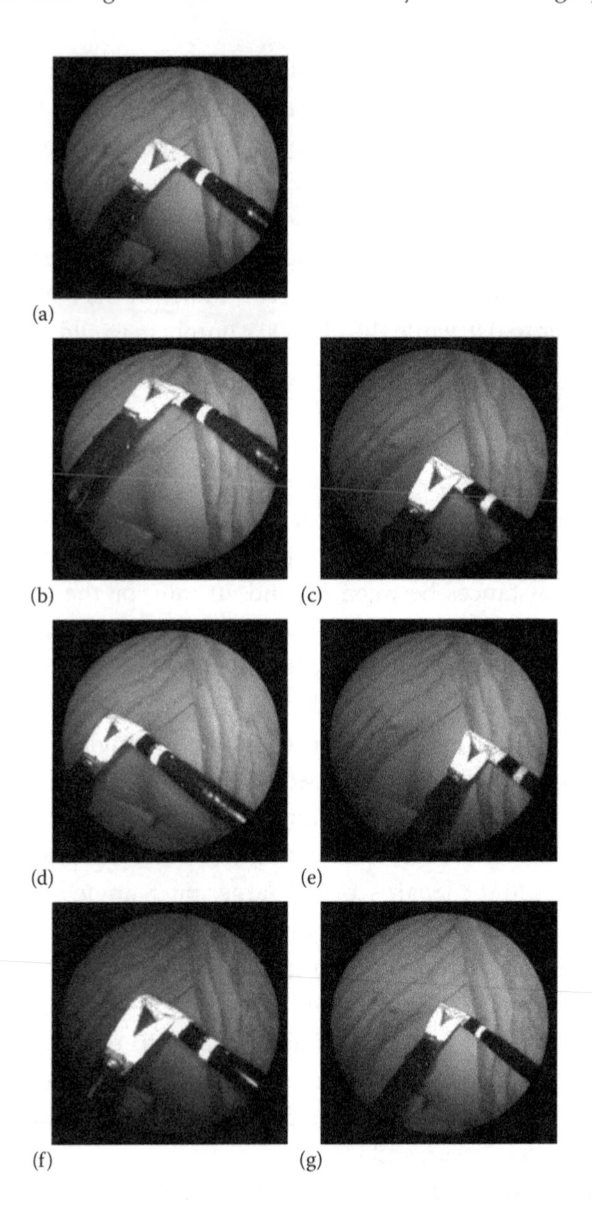

FIGURE 3.23 The seven orientations of overlapping double-tool gestures. (a) Middle; (b) up; (c) down; (d) left; (e) right; (f) near; (g) far.

smaller negative pitch angle, larger negative pitch angle, positive yaw angle, negative yaw angle, and random orientations, which are 90%, 100%, 70%, 100%, 80%, 70%, 100%, and 80%, respectively. This gesture is better recognized at natural, positive roll angle, smaller negative pitch angle, and negative yaw angle orientations. The overall recognition rate for the closed

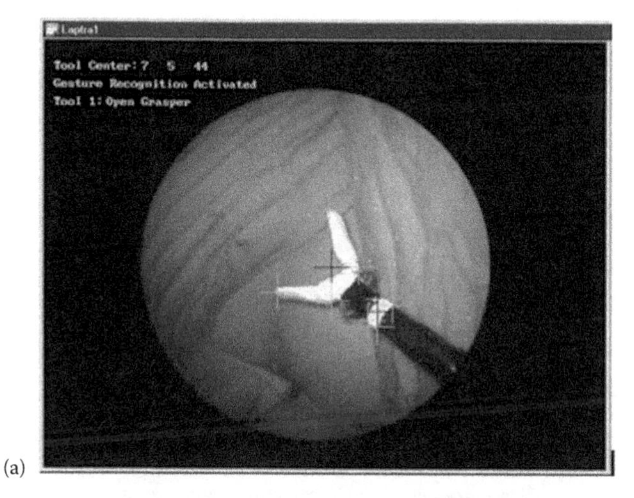

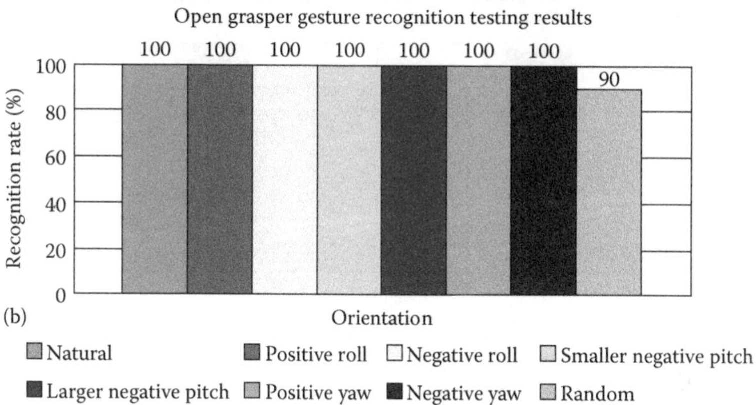

FIGURE 3.24 (a) An example of an open surgical grasper being recognized; (b) its associated recognition rates.

grasper gesture is 86.25%. Although the overall recognition rate of this gesture is not as high as the recognition rate for the open grasper gesture, the closed grasper gesture is still a reliable gesture, as it can be recognized almost nine out of every 10 times.

Figure 3.26 shows the closed surgical scissors gesture being recognized with the presence of the surgical grasper and the corresponding recognition rates. These are for the natural, positive roll angle, negative roll angle, smaller negative pitch angle, larger negative pitch angle, positive yaw angle, negative yaw angle, and random orientations are 90%, 80%, 100%, 100%, 100%, 70%, 70%, and 80%, respectively. The recognition rates are lower at either positive or negative yaw angles. Overall, the

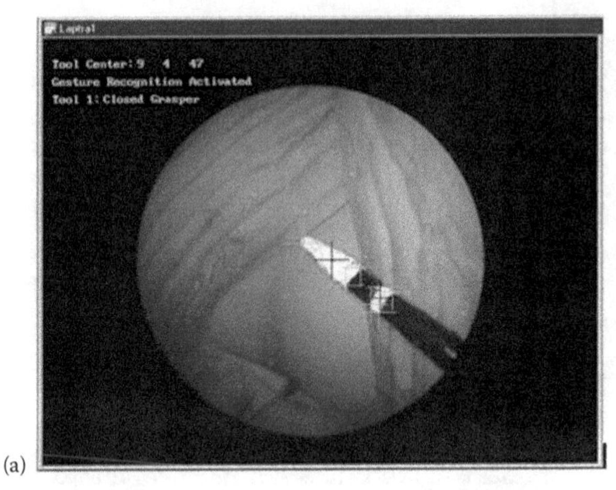

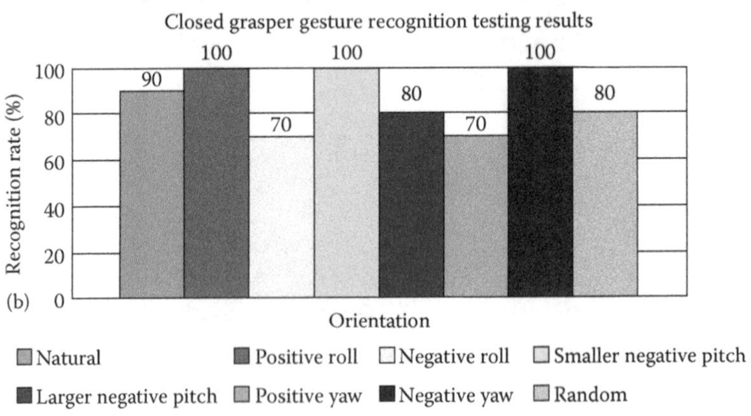

FIGURE 3.25 (a) An example of a closed surgical grasper being recognized; (b) its associated recognition rates for various orientations.

closed scissors gesture can be recognized at a rate of 86.25%, making it a reliable tool gesture.

Despite being one of the basic single-tool gestures, the 48.75% overall recognition rate for the open scissors gesture shown in Figure 3.27 is far lower than the other three single-tool gestures. The recognition rate for the natural, positive roll angle, negative roll angle, smaller negative pitch angle, larger negative pitch angle, positive yaw angle, negative yaw angle, and random orientations are 20%, 70%, 90%, 50%, 0%, 50%, 60%, and 50%, respectively. The recognition rates are extremely poor at the natural position (20%) and large negative pitch angle (0%). However, the recognition rates are significantly higher when the open scissors gesture is performed at either a positive roll angle (70%) or a negative roll angle (90%).

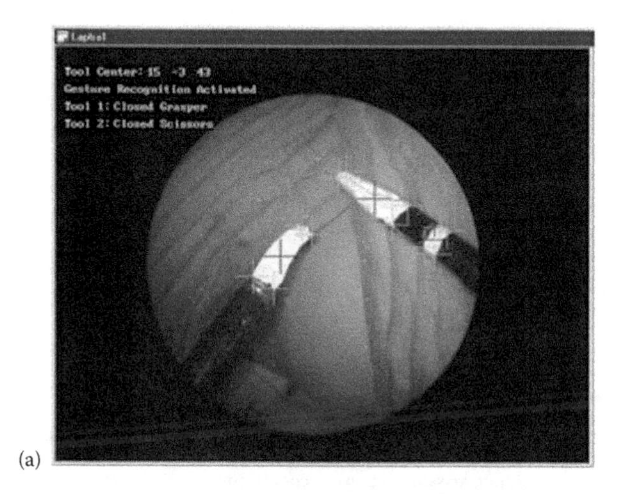

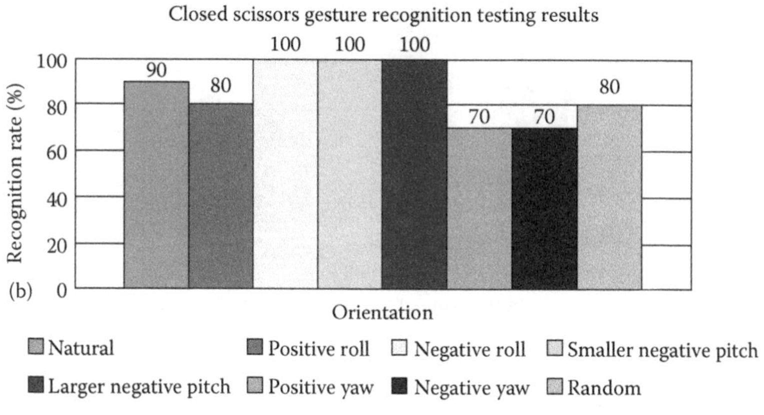

FIGURE 3.26 (a) An example of closed surgical scissors being recognized in a natural configuration; (b) their associated recognition rates for various orientations.

The open scissors gesture is often misidentified as the triangle gesture shown in Figure 3.12j, resulting in a low overall recognition rate. One possible contributing factor to the low recognition rate is that the open scissors are part of the triangle gesture. Consequently, the feature quantities extracted from an open scissors gesture may confuse the NN because they are similar to those of a triangle gesture. The higher recognition rates at positive and negative roll angles also support this assumption. When the open scissors gesture is performed at a roll angle, the feature quantities extracted would be less similar to those of a triangle gesture that contains open scissors at natural orientation.

Figure 3.28 shows the overlapping double-tool cross gesture and the recognition rates for the middle, up, down, left, right, near, far, and

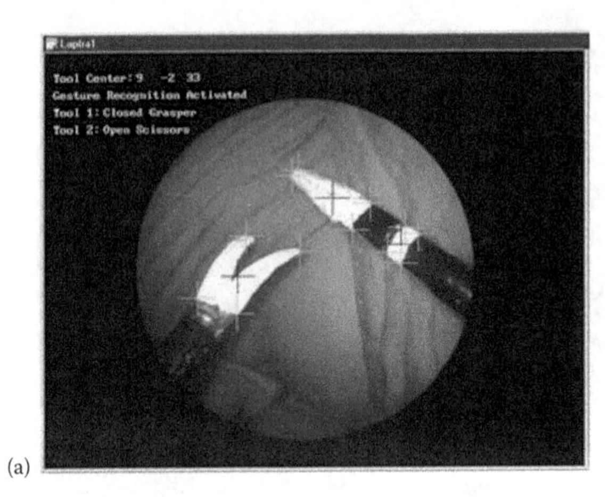

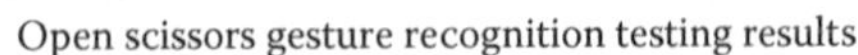

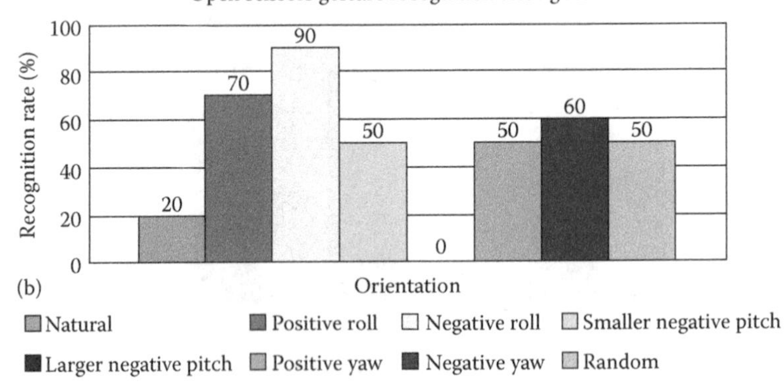

FIGURE 3.27 (a) An example of open surgical scissors being recognized; (b) their associated recognition rates for various orientations.

random orientations, which are 50%, 70%, 30%, 60%, 40%, 40%, 80%, and 70%, respectively. The overall recognition rate of this gesture is 55%. The recognition rates are above average at the up, left, and away orientations. At 80%, the recognition at the away orientation is the highest of all seven orientations, which means the cross gesture is actually better recognized when it is performed further away from the laparoscope.

The overall recognition rate of the triangle gesture shown in Figure 3.29 is 38.75%, and the corresponding recognition rates for the middle, up, down, left, right, close, away, and random orientations are 20%, 40%, 30%, 40%, 50%, 50%, 40%, and 40%, respectively. The recognition rates are higher at the right and close orientations, where the scissors are in the middle of the image and are better illuminated.

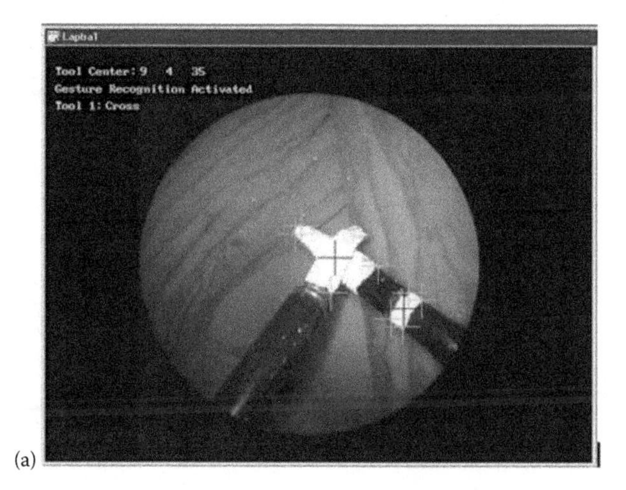

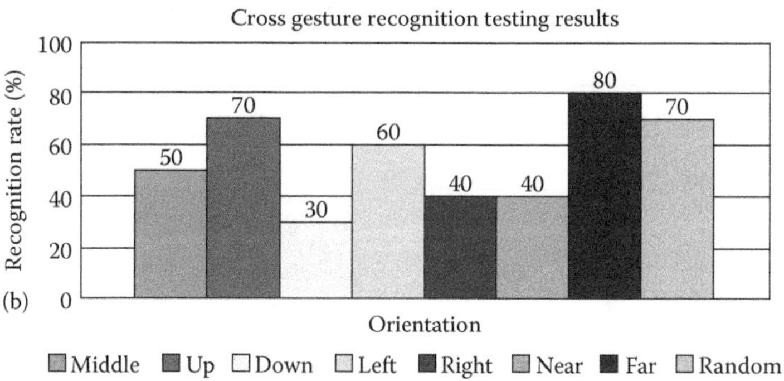

FIGURE 3.28 (a) An example of a cross configuration of surgical tools being recognized; (b) the associated recognition rates at various positions with respect to the endoscope.

The double triangle gesture is the hardest to perform and is unrecognizable, with the result that the recognition rates for all the orientations are 0%. It is usually recognized as the single-tool open grasper gesture. Visually, the double triangle gesture consists of an open grasper gesture and an open scissors gesture, so it is not surprising that the double triangle gesture is often recognized as an open grasper gesture.

Overall, the overlapping double-tool gestures are more difficult to perform than single-tool gestures, so their recognition rates are expected to be lower than those of single-tool gestures. When performing an overlapping double-tool gesture, sometimes it is difficult to manipulate the two surgical tools to form a single blob. Sometimes the positions of the two surgical tools with respect to each other can be too far off from any one

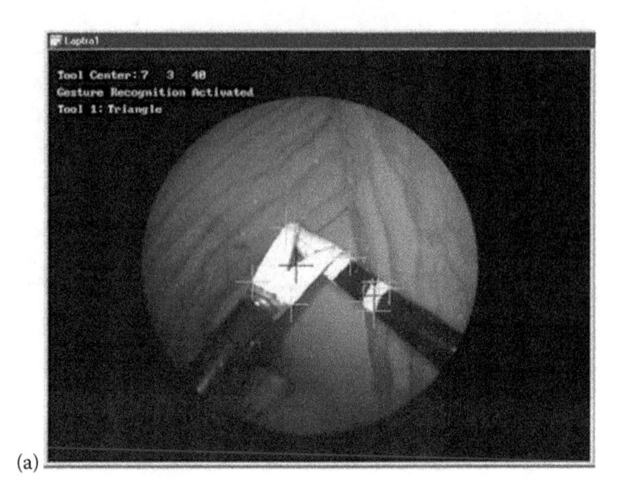

(a)

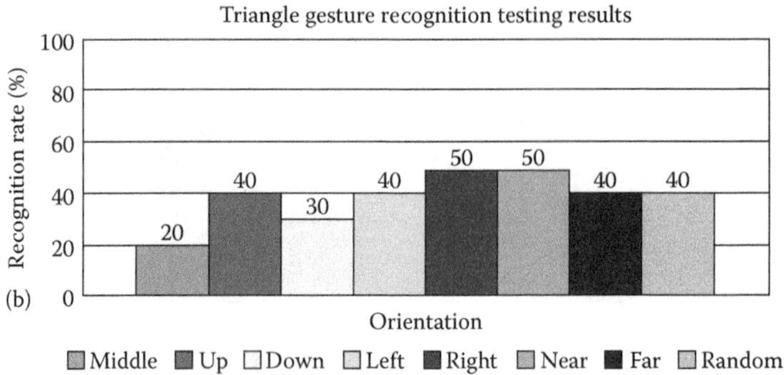

(b)

FIGURE 3.29 (a) An example of a triangular gesture being recognized; (b) the associated recognition rates at various positions with respect to the endoscope.

of the designed tool gestures in Figure 3.12. Consequently, the performed overlapping double-tool gestures are misidentified either as two single-tool gestures, or as the closest tool gesture the NN interprets them to be.

In addition, for an overlapping double-tool gesture to be recognized, the two tool tips are supposed to overlap and form only a single blob. This requirement is often not easy to achieve due to the shadows of the surgical tools. In some cases, the shadows can actually help in obtaining the depth information. However, in our case, the shadow of one surgical tool cast on the other will often break up the single blob into two. As a result, the overlapping double-tool gestures are often misidentified as two single-tool gestures, which further lower the recognition rates.

The overall surgical tool gesture recognition rates for the seven single-tool and overlapping double-tool gestures are shown in Figure 3.30.

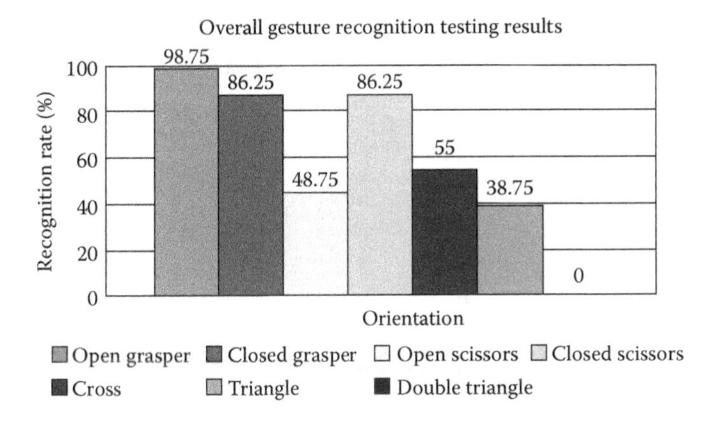

FIGURE 3.30 Overall surgical tool gesture recognition rates for the seven single-tool and overlapping double-tool gestures.

The recognition rates for the open grasper gesture, closed grasper gesture, open scissors gesture, closed scissors gesture, cross gesture, triangle gesture, and double triangle gesture are 98.75%, 86.25%, 48.75%, 86.25%, 55%, 38.78%, and 0%, respectively. The open grasper, closed grasper, and closed scissors gestures can all be recognized at over 86%, which suggests that they are reliable tool gestures. Although the overall recognition rate of the open scissors gesture is only 48.75%, it can still be recognized about eight out of 10 times when the gesture is performed at either positive or negative roll angles. Therefore, this gesture can still be considered a reliable tool gesture, as long as the operator keeps in mind that the gesture has to be performed with a roll angle.

The overlapping double-tool gestures are not as recognizable as the single-tool gestures. At 55%, the recognition rate of the cross gesture is barely over 50%. However, when performed at a distance from a laparoscope, this gesture can actually be recognized at 80%, which is a respectable percentage. The triangle and double triangle gestures, recognized at 38.75% and 0% overall, respectively, are the two gestures with the lowest recognition rates. The tool gesture recognition function has to be improved to raise their recognition rates in the future for these two tool gestures to be useful.

Table 3.3 shows the confusion matrix of the tool gesture recognition function. For example, the second row shows that the open grasper tool gesture is correctly recognized 79 times out of 80 trials. Only one trial is misidentified as the double-triangle tool gesture. The confusion matrix shows that most of the tool gestures are misidentified as the triangle gesture for a significant amount of trials, suggesting that the recognition

TABLE 3.3 Tool Gesture Recognition Confusion Matrix

	Recognized						
Performed	**Open Grasper**	**Closed Grasper**	**Open Scissors**	**Closed Scissors**	**Cross**	**Triangle**	**Double Triangle**
Open grasper	79	0	0	0	0	0	1
Closed grasper	0	69	0	0	2	9	0
Open scissors	0	0	39	10	0	31	0
Closed scissors	0	0	2	69	2	7	0
Cross	3	0	0	0	44	33	0
Triangle	0	5	7	9	28	31	0
Double triangle	46	0	0	0	5	29	0

rates of those tool gestures, especially the open scissors and cross gestures, could be improved by removing the triangle tool gesture.

Although the illumination brightness as tested is 35 lx, the gesture recognition still works quite well when the brightness is set as low as 25 lx. When the brightness is increased, the gesture recognition works well up until about 50 lx. However, it is not recommended to turn up the brightness too high because the background objects would be too bright and would pass the threshold value, causing confusions in the target tool segmentation process. In addition, the tool gestures are suggested to be performed as close to the center of the image as possible, where the illumination is strong and even, and without extreme roll, pitch, or yaw angles.

Overall, the high recognition rate of single-tool gestures and non-overlapping double-tool gestures show that the surgical tool gesture recognition function can be used as a practical and reliable SCI. With the development of a more accurate tool gesture classifier that could classify overlapping double-tool gestures more accurately and recognize more different surgical tool gestures, this function would definitely impact the evolution of the surgical SCI.

DESIGN OF SURGEON–COMPUTER INTERFACES

In this section, applications of the surgical tool gesture and motion recognitions are explored in order to design and develop various notions for SCIs. For example, a hybrid SCI is proposed that utilizes the combined recognition methods (Payandeh et al. 2012). Here, the surgical tool gesture recognition function can be triggered by manually pressing a switch on the handle of surgical tool and can be terminated by performing a cross-tool gesture. The tool motion recognition function can be triggered by performing an open grasper and it can be terminated by either performing a closed grasper gesture or reaching the maximum number of motion trajectory sample points.

In one implementation of hybrid SCI, the surgeon is only required to use one tool gesture and one tool motion to access three different types of medical information and images. For example, the open grasper tool gesture and the loop tool motion (circular motion) can be selected.

Here, various approaches are proposed that can be followed in order to trigger, use, and terminate tool gesture and motion recognition:

a. *Interface activation*: The tool gesture and motion recognition SCI is activated by keeping the scissors stationary within a shaded activation area at the bottom of the camera image, as shown in Figure 3.31, for 3 s. The system uses the 2D projection of the center of the scissors tool tip blob to determine if the scissors are within the activation area.

b. *Function selection*: When the hybrid SCI based on tool gesture and motion recognition is activated, four graphically overlaid function buttons are displayed on the live endoscopic video stream. The surgeon can use the surgical grasper to choose one of the functions by performing an open grasper tool gesture within the overlaid graphical areas. When an open grasper gesture is recognized, the system verifies if the center of the tool gesture blob is within the areas of the function buttons.

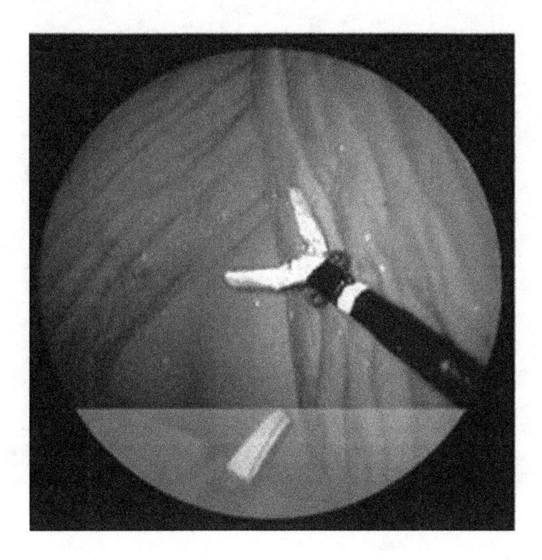

FIGURE 3.31 The activation area of surgical tool gesture recognition.

Figure 3.32 shows the *Display MRI* function being selected. A message pops up in the middle of the camera image asking for user confirmation. This figure also shows other overlaid menu options that can be selected by the surgeon, which include the *Display XRAY*, *Display CAT*, and *EXIT* functions (Figure 3.32b).

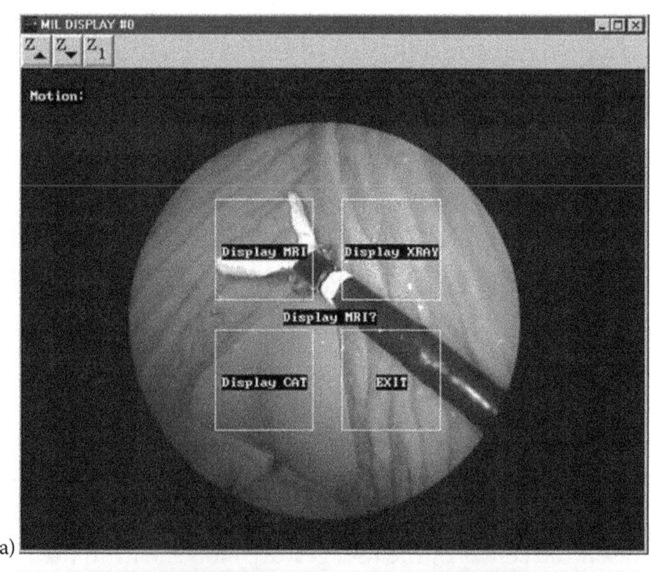

(a)

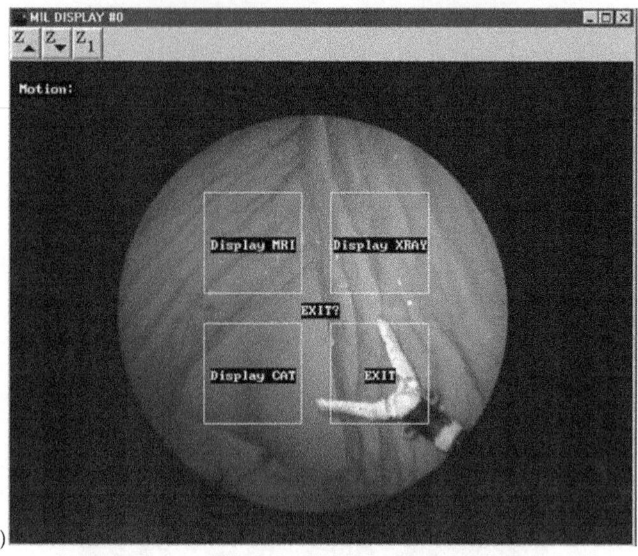

(b)

FIGURE 3.32 Example of a SCI for (a) accessing and (b) terminating medical information using an open tool position.

c. *Function selection confirmation*: To confirm the function selection, the surgeon can perform a loop tool motion within the next 2 s. Upon confirmation, the system prints a confirmation message, as shown in Figure 3.33a, and executes the function. Any tool motions other than the loop tool motion would deny the confirmation as

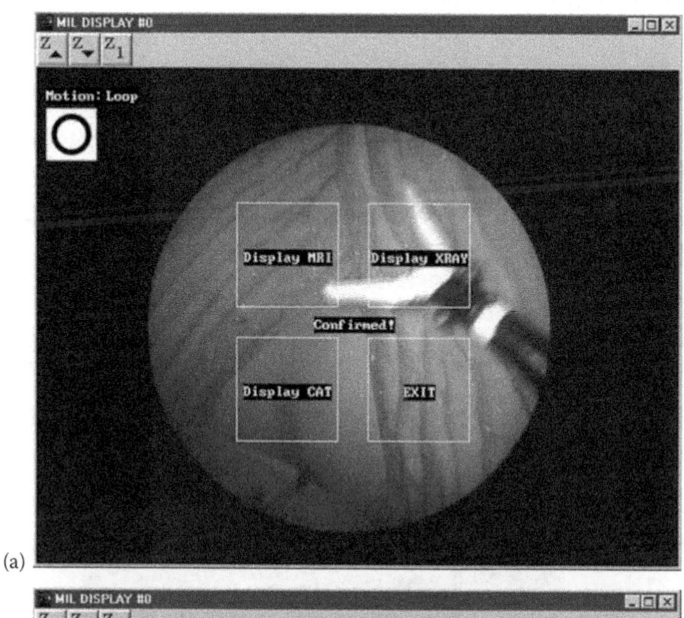

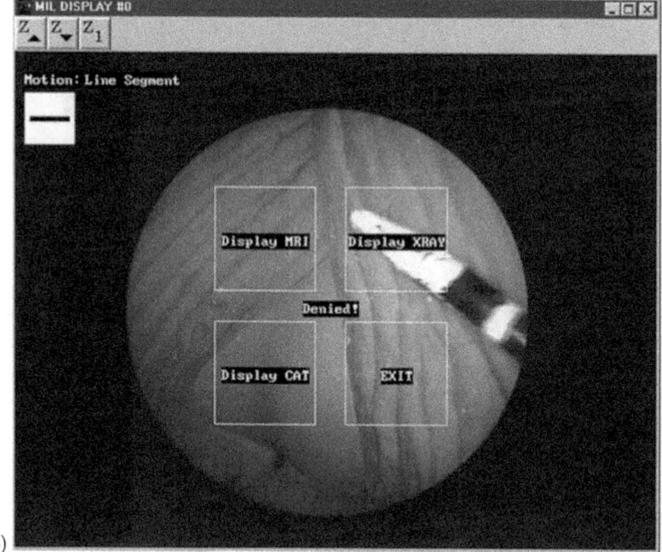

FIGURE 3.33 Examples of menu functions being (a) selected and (b) confirmed by making the required motion of the surgical tool.

shown in Figure 3.33b. The user can select another function again when the selected function is either executed or denied.

d. *Exit*: To exit the interface, the user will only need to select the *EXIT* function by performing an open grasper tool gesture and then performing a loop tool motion to confirm.

Another example of a SCI is shown in Figure 3.34a. In this implementation and in order to avoid accidental activation of the overlaid augmented mode, the formed gesture needs to be held for 1 s to be recognized by the system. When a gesture is recognized, the field of view of the endoscope, except the middle section, is divided into four regions: *Open CT*, *Open X-Ray*, *Open MRI*, and *Exit*, which are overlaid on the field of view of the endoscope.

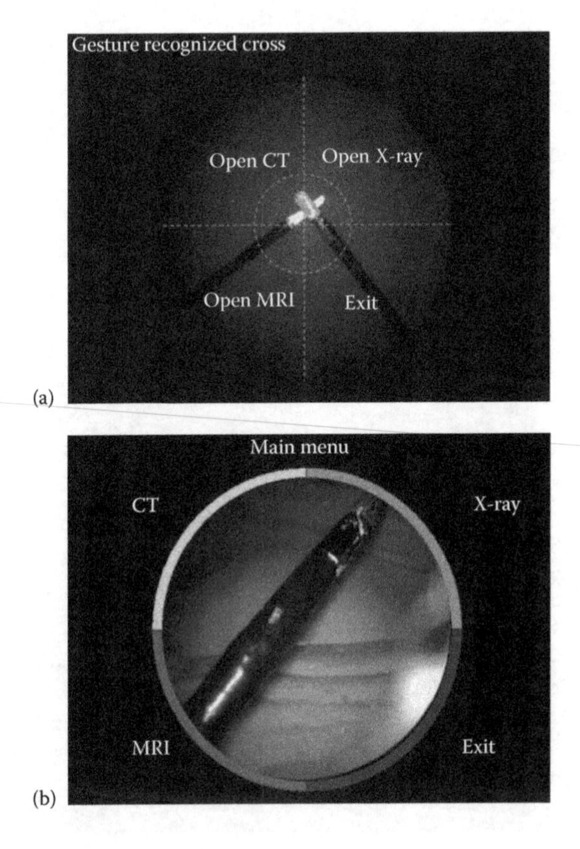

FIGURE 3.34 Examples of an SCI: (a) using surgical tools to form a cross gesture, an overlaid menu is activated; (b) an example of a ring menu formed around the endoscopic view.

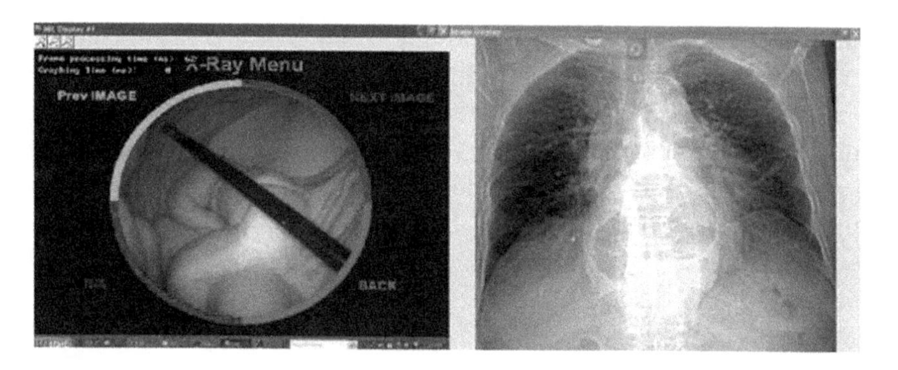

FIGURE 3.35 In the *X-Ray Menu* selection mode, the surgeon can choose the previous or next image or go back to the main menu.

Another example of SCI design is to display a narrow ring around the field of view of the endoscope (Figure 3.34b). The surgeon operates in a graphically overlaid environment from the beginning of the surgery. This ring basically acts as an option menu that allows the surgeon to choose a specific function and have access to a particular medical record of the patient. For example, this ring can be divided into four different regions: *CT*, *X-RAY*, *MRI*, and *EXIT*. Once a menu option is selected, the submenu overlaid ring is shown (Figure 3.35), which can offer the surgeon more options for manipulating the medical information.

SUMMARY

This chapter has presented applications of visual tracking and recognition using predefined markers that can be placed on the surgical tool or configured by the tool. Using the calibration parameters of the endoscope, it was shown how the tracking information of the surgical tool with respect to the endoscope reference frame can be obtained. It was shown that, while it is possible to determine the depth information of the surgical tool with respect to the endoscopic frame, it also affects the scale factor in the planar direction. An interpolation function was developed, whereby it is possible to compute the true spatial information of the surgical tool with respect to the endoscopic frame. The computed tracking information of the surgical tool was compared by a measure of ground truth and also with the use of external measuring devices. It was shown that the proposed method shows good performance when compared with the ground truth. Various gestures of surgical tool tips that can be made by the surgeon were used in defining various common visual features. These features can be extracted through the proposed image-processing methods, which can further be classified and stored. Using the notion of machine learning through the implementation of artificial NN, the performance of the gesture recognition system was shown through various examples. Next, it was shown how the results of the tracking and recognition of the motion and gestures of the surgical tool can be used as an approach for developing SCIs. Examples of such interfaces through the design of overlaid graphical menus were introduced. In these examples, the surgeon can access medical images and information through placement of the surgical tool and/or by performing a given gesture within the endoscopic view.

CHAPTER 4

Markerless Tracking: Gaussian Approach

The field of markerless image tracking has been gaining popularity in many application areas. These include attempts in fields such as movement tracking (Dai and Payandeh 2013), statistical-based tracking for visual servoing (Marchand et al. 2005), and in extensions to principal component analysis for learning-based tracking (Ross et al. 2008). Each of these algorithms is designed and tailored in order to satisfy the requirements and constraints associated with the properties of the tracked objects and the environments in which they are being tracked. This chapter presents studies in the field of markerless visual tracking of surgical tools in the minimally invasive surgery (MIS) environment.

Initially, some preliminary analysis of the motion history image (MHI) approach, which is one of the most basic approaches for markerless visual tracking, is presented (Lu and Payandeh 2008). Through the application of the MHI approach, it is possible to define a region of interest (ROI) around moving objects (e.g., surgical tools) and to extract their relative size and orientation in the endoscopic field of view. Next, feature-based tracking methods are presented. Unlike the method of the previous chapter, these approaches do not rely on any specific markers attached to the surgical tools. These methods are based on the assumption of linearity of the dynamic models representing the movements of the surgical tools. In addition, these methods are able to track the moving target (e.g., surgical tool) in the presence of noise in the movements and measurements, which can be represented by Gaussian distribution.

OVERVIEW OF MOVEMENT TRACKING USING MOTION HISTORY IMAGES

This approach uses image frame differences in order to create an MHI (Bradski and Davis 2002). This history of motion can also be represented by a function in terms of motion sequences. An MHI is an image that is obtained by compressing the image–time volume onto a single image. The intensity values in the MHI indicate the time at which a pixel last registered a motion or the presence of an object. An MHI captures the essence of the underlying motion pattern for the surgical tool by taking the difference of *N* frames simultaneously over the last *N* time steps. By analyzing the motion, we can extract information such as the direction of motion and velocity of the surgical tool.

The MHI is updated after each sampling period by adding the newly detected frame difference. For example, given *N* frames, simple frame difference subtraction can be applied. Then the *N* image silhouettes are converted into a single template. Every time a new frame is captured, the existing silhouettes are weighted to be less important, such that having brighter MHI values depicts more recent motion. The new silhouette is overlaid based on this weight, and, in this case, the binary intensity can be used for further image processing.

Figure 4.1b shows an example of an MHI representing a tool. The more recent movements have greater intensity than the past events. Once the MHI is obtained, motion gradients can be efficiently calculated by convolution with separable Sobel filters in the x and y directions of the image plane (Bradski and Davis 2002). The motion gradient along the x and y directions, F_x and F_y, are defined as

$$F_x = \frac{1}{8}\begin{bmatrix} -1 & 0 & 1 \\ -2 & 0 & 2 \\ -1 & 0 & 1 \end{bmatrix} \quad F_y = \frac{1}{8}\begin{bmatrix} -1 & -2 & -1 \\ 0 & 0 & 0 \\ 1 & 2 & 1 \end{bmatrix} \tag{4.1}$$

Given the resultant magnitude of gradients at the pixel location (x, y) as $F_x(x, y)$ and $F_y(x, y)$, the gradient orientation can be defined as

$$\phi(x,y) = \arctan\frac{F_y(x,y)}{F_x(x,y)} \tag{4.2}$$

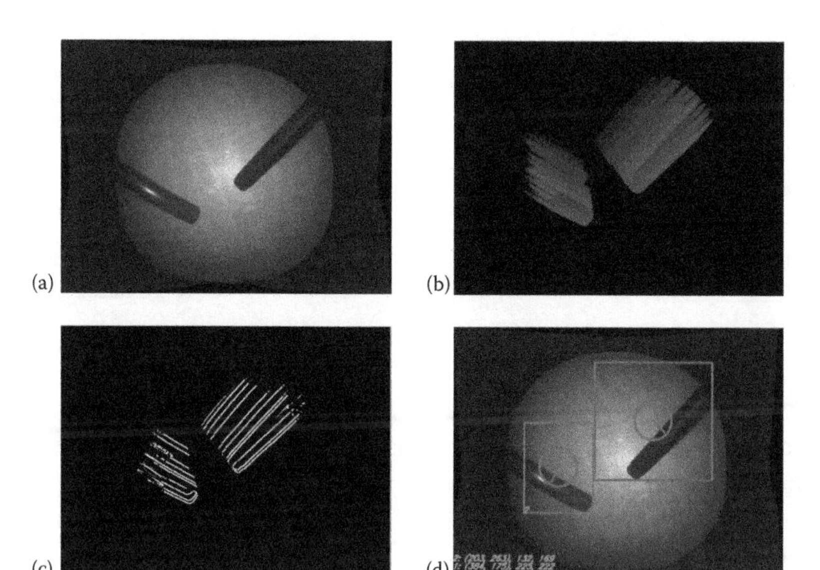

FIGURE 4.1 Tracking the surgical tool using MHI: (a) the original input frame of the tool; (b) the MHI of the frame; (c) the calculated motion gradient of the image; (d) the detected bounding box and direction of motion (circular dial) obtained by analyzing MHI.

and the magnitude of the gradient as

$$\mathrm{Mag}(x,y)=\sqrt{F_x^2(x,y)+F_y^2(x,y)} \tag{4.3}$$

Through the result of this computation (Figure 4.1c), motion features can be extracted to varying scales. For example, it is possible to track different surgical tools simultaneously and to initialize and label them during the visual tracking.

Once the MHI is obtained, a pixel dilation and region-growing method is applied in order to remove any unwanted noise. The motion is then segmented relative to the object boundaries in order to determine the motion tendency of each tool at a given instance (Figure 4.1d). Figure 4.2 shows the basic flow diagram associated with the process of Figure 4.1 (Lu and Payandeh 2008).

Given the ROI of the tracking target, the tip of the surgical tool can be detected easily. The tip is estimated to be the point of intersection between the middle line of the tool and the bounding box (Figure 4.3). The middle line always intersects with two edges, generating two intersection points.

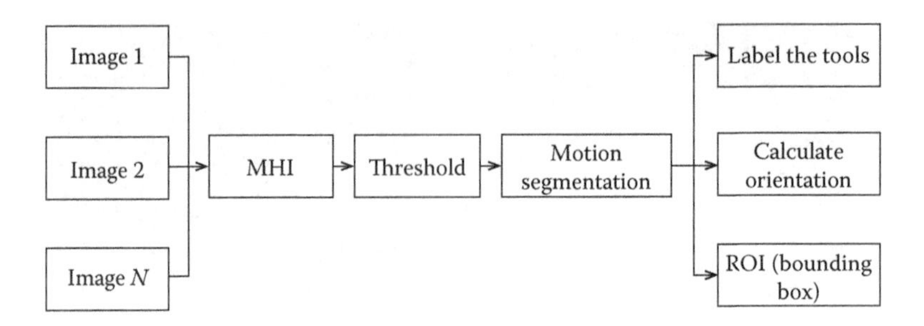

FIGURE 4.2 MHI motion detection flow chart.

To choose a valid tip location, we made the assumption that the tip is always closer to the center of the view (more details about the method for detecting the tip of the surgical tool can be found in the following sections).

Figure 4.4 shows examples of typical image frames—for example, frames 12, 51, 52, and 138 of the MHI method. In frame 52, because of the fast motion of the tool, the bounding box generated in the MHI is bigger than the actual border. However, the bounding box can always be used in order to define the maximum upper-limit bounding of the tool. Thus, it

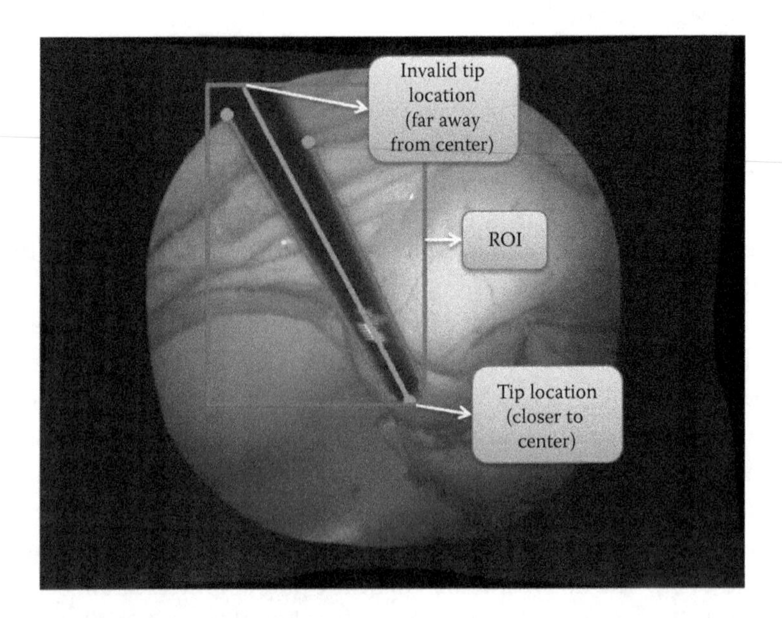

FIGURE 4.3 Example of surgical tool tip extraction given the ROI of the tracking target.

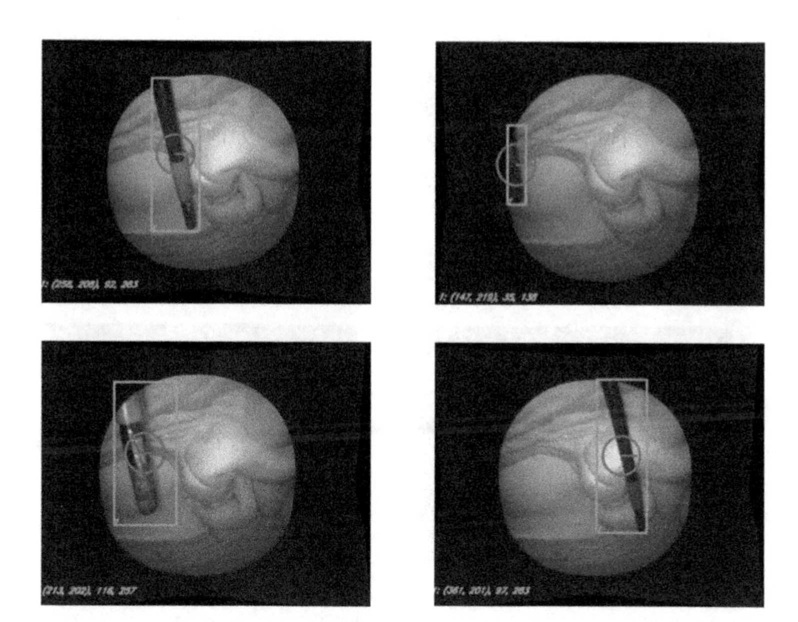

FIGURE 4.4 MHI results when the motion of a single surgical tool is being tracked in the view of a stationary endoscope. The rectangles represent the bounding box (ROI) of the whole object and the circular dial represents the current directional flow of motion.

can be utilized for defining the ROI in the initialization phase of the tracking methods. For example, the segmented MHI and ROI can be utilized as initial templates for the Kalman filter (KF) algorithm for tracking surgical tools (see the following sections).

In summary, the MHI is a computationally fast algorithm for tracking multiple targets, and it offers a basis for simple surgical tool tip extraction. However, when several tools are moving or crossing each other's paths, the motion segmentation fails to detect the separate regions for each of the bounding boxes (as shown in Figure 4.5). Another drawback is that when the tool is moving fast, the ROI is larger than the tool's actual bounding box, causing inaccurate estimation of the tool tip location (as shown in Figure 4.6).

FEATURE-BASED TRACKING

The purpose of the tracking algorithm is to calculate the position and orientation of the surgical tool in 3-D space. Assuming the tool has a uniform cylindrical shape with a known physical diameter, information about the location of its edges and the position of its tool tip is needed

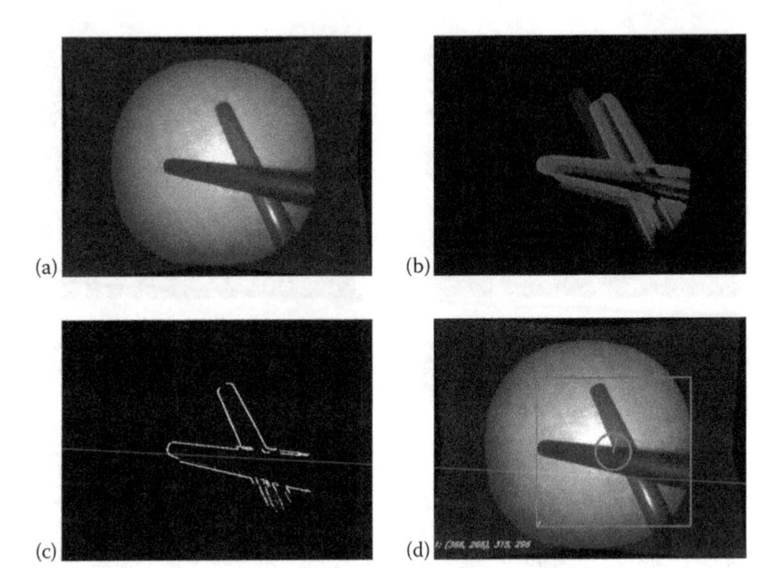

FIGURE 4.5 Failed example of tracking multiple surgical tools using MHI when the tools cross each other's paths: (a) the original input frame; (b) the MHI of the frame; (c) the computed motion gradient of the image; (d) the detected bounding box and estimate of the direction of movement (circular dial).

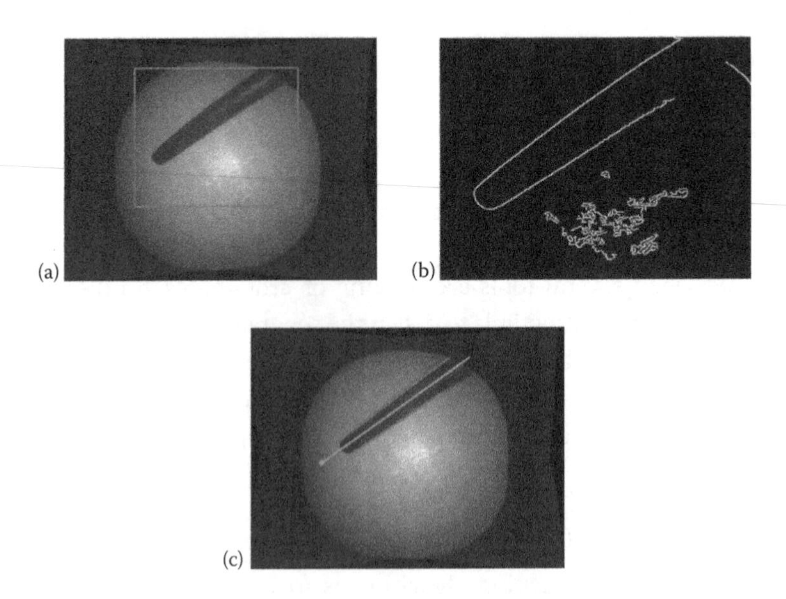

FIGURE 4.6 Surgical tool tip extraction given the ROI detected using MHI: (a) the ROI extracted using MHI; (b) Canny edge detection applied within ROI; (c) the extracted edges of the surgical tool, middle line, and the tip.

at least in order to characterize the spatial information of the tool in the 3-D space. The MHI-based tracking approach can be extended in order to resolve the 3-D reconstruction of tools without combining the model-based information—namely, the edges and tip.

A robust 3-D tracking system is proposed in this chapter, combining both the stochastic approach and feature-based recognition. Our assumption here is that the endoscope system is stationary during the tracking process and it is also calibrated. It is also assumed that information about the physical size and dimensions of the surgical tool is available. As mentioned previously, tracking the surgical tool is a very challenging problem due to the following:

a. *Few textures on the instrument*: Most tracking algorithms use texture analysis to detect/track objects, which tends to be more robust and feasible. Without textures, few tracking algorithms can be adapted and extended for tracking surgical tools.

b. *Scene dynamic of the surgical site*: The real surgical scene has a complex background, such as organs, tissues, multiple surgical tools, and so on, making recognition of the surgical instrument very challenging, especially for multiple-tool tracking. Another problem is light reflection on the scene, which makes recognition even more challenging.

c. *Partial occlusion and fast movement of the surgical instruments*: The surgical instrument can be contaminated by blood or partially occluded by smoke during surgical operation. Moreover, the fast movement of the surgical instrument blurs the images, causing a loss of tracking.

d. *Surgical performance constraints*: The tracking must be accurate and fast enough (10–60 fps) to be applied during the surgical procedure.

This chapter explores the application of the KF approach to extend the robustness of the tracking system and at the same time support multiple surgical tool tracking. The chapter also presents the design of the edge/tip extraction module, which offers a solution to tool occlusion problems by using the edges of the surgical tools as visual features instead of markers. Finally, the 3-D reconstruction module allows us to take advantage of the single camera to map 2-D information to 3-D.

Overview of the Feature-Based Tracking Algorithm

Motion-based approaches such as the MHI method are able to extract the motion of the target. However, these methods are not capable of extending the tracking and reconstruction of surgical tools into 3-D space. The reason is that a full geometrical reconstruction needs to include not only the position of the tip but also the two edges of the assumed cylindrical shape of the rigid surgical tool. Here we propose an algorithm that solves the 3-D tracking problems and offers both 2-D tracking and a 3-D reconstruction module. Various comparisons are also presented in order to show the advantages of the proposed method over the previous tracking algorithms.

The proposed visual tracking algorithm is different from the tracking method shown in the previous chapter. This method uses shape and feature analysis instead of using the assigned markers on the surgical tool. An overview of the proposed tracking algorithm (as shown in Figure 4.7) is as follows: The program obtains the 2-D position of the edge and tip of the surgical tool as an initial input for KF tracking. Once the initialization is complete, the tracking algorithm initiates. First it handles the preprocessing of the image frames. Then it tracks the tool orientation vector (middle line of the tool) and updates its Kalman state. If the tool is lost during the tracking, the system reinitializes its state; otherwise, the

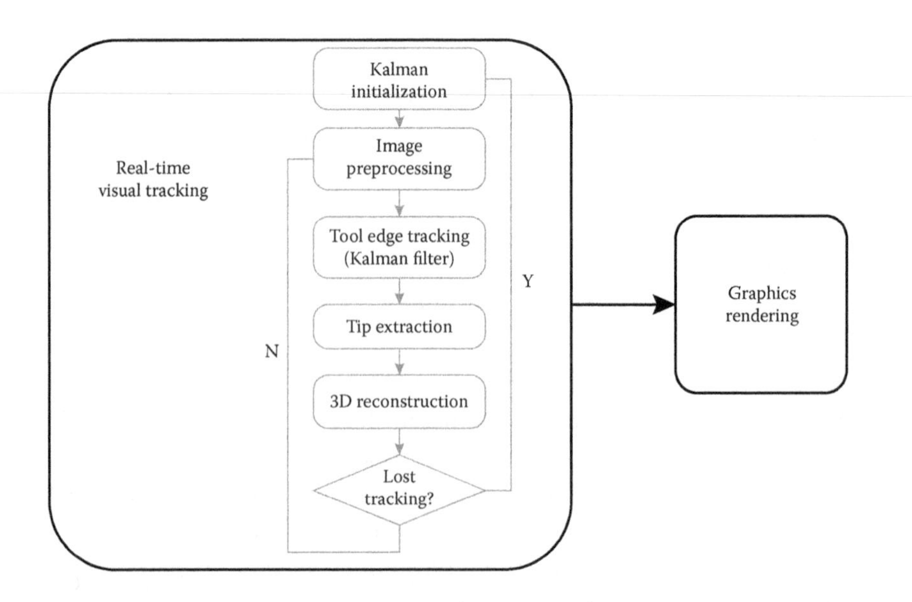

FIGURE 4.7 Visual tracking module and flowchart.

system continues its tracking. Based on the orientation estimation of the middle line, edges that do not belong to the tool are filtered. Then, the tool tip extraction module extracts the tip position based on the middle line of the tool. Finally, the 3-D reconstruction module takes the two valid edges and the tip position as the input and geometrically reconstructs the position and orientation of the tool in 3-D space. The remainder of this section will further highlight some of the details about the proposed method.

Two-Dimensional Tracking of Surgical Tools

In order to calculate the 3-D pose of the tool, its 2-D information has to be extracted first—namely, the edges and tip of the tool. As stated, the tracking algorithm has three major modules. The first module handles the initialization and preprocessing of the image frames. The second module is the KF module, whose purpose is to track the middle line of the tool and filter out the edges (coming from the background or other objects) that don't belong to the tool. The last module is to extract the 2-D edges and tip location. The module is processed in the order of Canny edge detection, the Hough transform, edge postprocessing, and tip extraction. Canny edge detection, the Hough transform, and edge postprocessing serve the purpose of edge extraction. After the edges of the tool are extracted, the middle line of the tool can be calculated. Since the tip is lying along the middle line of the tool, which is assumed to be rigid in shape and symmetrical, the tip can be identified at the end using the tip of the surgical tool. The following section will elaborate each of the modules and their functionality.

Kalman Filter

In order to reconstruct the configuration of the surgical tool in 3-D, the edges and tip position have to be calculated in each frame. The simplest approach for such detection is through the use of Canny edge and corner detection. However, this approach is not robust in a variant environment where light reflection and partial object occlusion exist. Moreover, edge detection can fail when there is more than one tool present in the surgical scene, which results in multiple edges that cannot be properly labeled. As an alternative, the KF is explored in order to address such tracking problems. This top-down tracking approach is able to estimate and track the current frame based on the previous one even when the tool is partially occluded or disappears from view for a short period of time.

The KF has long been regarded as the optimal solution to many tracking and data prediction problems. The purpose of filtering is to extract the required information from a signal. It is recursive, so that new measurements can be processed as they arrive. The dynamical system is represented using a state-space model where the unknown state is predicted based on the system model or estimated based on observations/measurements.

The KF is based on linear dynamical systems that can be represented in discrete domains. For example, the KF addresses the problem of estimating the state $X \in R^n$ of a process that is governed by the following linear stochastic difference equation:

$$X_t = AX_{t-1} + BU_{t-1} + W_{t-1} \tag{4.4}$$

with a measurement $Z \in R^m$ defined as

$$Z_t = MX_t + V_t \tag{4.5}$$

The random variables W_t and V_t represent the process and measurement noise, respectively. They are assumed to be independent (of each other), white, and with normal probability distributions (Gaussian):

$$p(W) \sim N(0,Q),\ p(V) \sim N(0,R) \tag{4.6}$$

Here, it is assumed that the process noise covariance Q and measurement noise covariance R matrices are constant.

The $n \times n$ matrix A in Equation 4.4 relates the state at the previous time step ($t-1$) to the state at the current step (t), in the absence of either a driving function or process noise. The $n \times 1$ matrix B relates the optional control input $U \in R^l$ to the state variable X. The $m \times n$ matrix M in Equation 4.5 relates the state to the measurement Z_t.

In the proposed tracking system, the Kalman state is modeled as the position and velocity of the middle line of the surgical tool. The position of the middle line (see Figure 4.8) is parameterized by its slope m and the axis intercept b of its projection onto the image plane. The rate of change of these variables is defined as the first derivative of the slope and y intercept. Thus, the state X in frame t is modeled as

$$X_t = \left[m, b, m', b'\right]^T \tag{4.7}$$

where the middle line is represented as

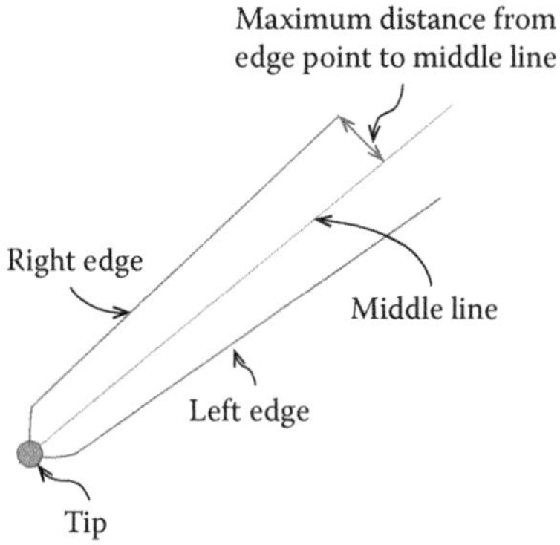

FIGURE 4.8 Surgical tool projection on the image plane.

$$y = mx + b \tag{4.8}$$

The state update equations can also be thought of as predictor equations, which in this case predict the location of the middle line for the current frame. The current frame t can be predicted from frame $t-1$ as

$$\begin{bmatrix} m_t \\ b_t \\ m'_t \\ b'_t \end{bmatrix} = \begin{bmatrix} 1 & 0 & 1 & 0 \\ 0 & 1 & 0 & 1 \\ 0 & 0 & 1 & 0 \\ 0 & 0 & 0 & 1 \end{bmatrix} \begin{bmatrix} m_{t-1} \\ b_{t-1} \\ m'_{t-1} \\ b'_{t-1} \end{bmatrix} + W_{t-1} \tag{4.9}$$

where:

W_{t-1} represents the process noise that can initiate from, for example, discontinuous motion of the surgical tool or modeling errors

(m_t, b_t) represents the middle line of the tool in the current frame

(m_{t-1}, b_{t-1}) represents the middle line of the tool in the previous frame

(m'_t, b'_t) and (m'_{t-1}, b'_{t-1}) denote the first derivatives of the slope and intercept parameters

The preceding definitions also imply that the rate of change of the parameters is kept constant throughout the transition; in another words, the positional parameter is linearly increasing or decreasing. The main assumption used in the preceding equation is that the impending velocity of the surgical tools can be considered within the normal operating range. The measurement model of the system is defined as

$$\begin{bmatrix} m_{\text{measure}_t} \\ b_{\text{measure}_t} \end{bmatrix} = \begin{bmatrix} 1 & 0 & 0 & 0 \\ 0 & 1 & 0 & 0 \end{bmatrix} \begin{bmatrix} m_t \\ b_t \\ m_t' \\ b_t' \end{bmatrix} + V_t \tag{4.10}$$

The system and measurement matrices A and M need to be initialized beforehand, similar to the model of the noise, including process noise W_t and measurement noise V_t. The noise variance is defined as

$$Q = \begin{bmatrix} 80 & 0 & 0 & 0 \\ 0 & 80 & 0 & 0 \\ 0 & 0 & 80 & 0 \\ 0 & 0 & 0 & 80 \end{bmatrix} \text{ and } R = \begin{bmatrix} 0.005 & 0.005 \\ 0.005 & 0.005 \end{bmatrix} \tag{4.11}$$

If the measurement noise covariance R is small, the final calculated state of the middle line position is nearly the same as the measurements obtained from image processing. Therefore, the magnitude of R is defined experimentally, which better reflects the measurement noise. By empirically testing different Q and R values, the estimation error covariance P_t and the Kalman gain K_t stabilize faster and remain unchanged (see the filter update algorithm given in the next section). Through experimental study, it was found that after three to six iterations, the error covariance remained in steady state, providing reliable selection of the noise covariance parameter.

Initialization and Preprocessing

The first problem is to detect and localize the middle line of the tool for the first frame, parameterized as m and b. Our initialization method is semi-automatic, which requires some initial preparation that can be done during the setup procedure of the surgical theater. The surgical tool is required to be placed in the endoscopic view. The imaging system detects the edges (those with maximum peaks in the Hough transform). The detected edges can be scattered and may not belong to the two edges of the surgical tool.

The image-processing system needs to be able to merge the edges to either the left or right part of the tool boundaries. The algorithm is summarized as follows:

a. Capture and load a frame of an image obtained from the video stream (Figure 4.10a).

b. Convert the colored image to gray scale so that the following Canny detector can be applied (Figure 4.10b).

c. Use the Canny detector to detect the edges of the image. Small segments of Canny output are directly discarded (Figure 4.10c).

d. Use the Hough transform to detect the straight lines appeared in the images. Several line segments are detected at the same time (Figure 4.10d).

e. Label the edge segments. Since the tool has two edges as a whole, each segment of the lines has to be labeled such that it belongs to either side of the edges. In order to label these lines, two sorting bins representing the two edges are initialized to store the line segments. The algorithm is performed as follows: The first line detected belongs to the first bin. Then the algorithm compares the second line with the first line; if the maximum distance between the end points of the second line to the first line (Figure 4.9) is larger than the threshold (in this case, 10 pixels), it is labeled to be in another bin—namely, another edge; otherwise, it belongs to the first bin. Similarly,

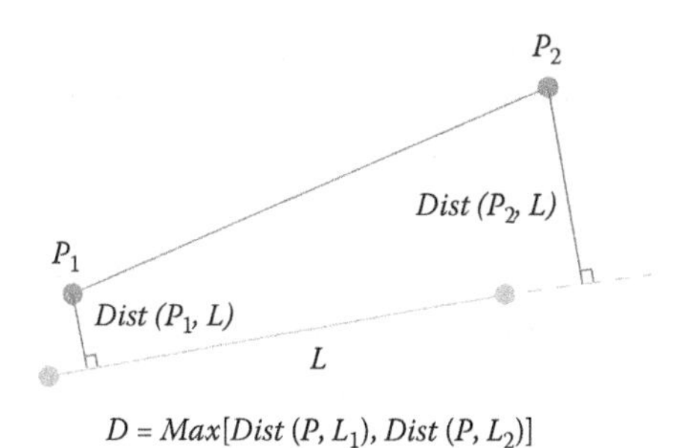

FIGURE 4.9 Illustration of the distance calculation between two edges. If the maximum distance of the end points of one line to the other line is less than the threshold ($D < Th$), it is assumed to be in the same bin; otherwise, it belongs to the other bin.

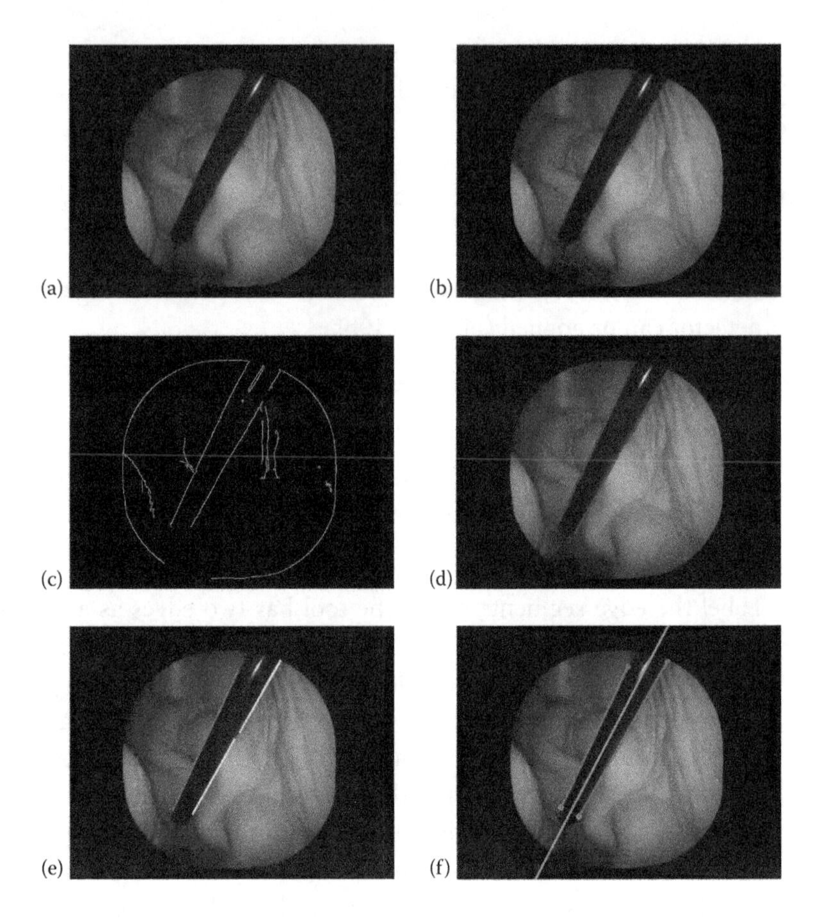

FIGURE 4.10 (a) Original input frame. (b) Converted gray image. (c) Output of Canny edge detector used for extracting edges of the tool. (d) Output of edge image detected using canny detector. (e) Edge segments classified into "left" and "right" edges. The lighter gray color segments belong to the "left" edge, and darker gray color ones are the "right" edge. (f) Edge segments merged together, forming two edges, a "left" edge and a "right" edge. A middle line between the two edges is then can be computed.

comparison is performed between the rest of the segments. Finally, each of the bins should store the corresponding line segments representing either side of the edges. To decide the distance between a random point in 2-D space, $P(x_0, y_0)$, and a line, the following equation is used:

$$Dist(P,\vec{L}) = \frac{|ax_0 + by_0 + c|}{\sqrt{a^2 + b^2}} \tag{4.12}$$

f. Once the edges have been classified into two bins, joining the line segments becomes the next step. For each bin or edge, the algorithm joins the leftmost point with the rightmost point, forming a single edge. Figure 4.10f shows the result of this method: the leftmost point and rightmost point are joined, forming a line. At this stage of computation, the two edges of the tool are extracted, denoted as $\vec{E}_1(m_1,b_1)$ and $\vec{E}_2(m_2,b_2)$. The middle line of the two edges then becomes:

$$\vec{E}(m,b) = \left(\frac{m_1 + m_2}{2}, \frac{b_1 + b_2}{2}\right) \tag{4.13}$$

Figure 4.10f shows the final result of the initialization, where the green line is the extracted middle line of the tool. The tracking algorithm remains initialized until the surgeon initiates the tracking using the activation mode button connected to the surgical handle.

Surgical Tool Tracking Using Standard Kalman Filtering

The KF is generally defined by a set of relationships providing an efficient recursively computational method to estimate the state of a process that can be defined as a linear dynamical system (Zarchan and Musoff 2009). The state of a process is expressed as a state vector that is composed of several unknown variables. These variables describe the instantaneous status of the target object. By using a series of measurements observed over time, the KF is able to estimate the current state vector.

As before, the state of the process in our case is the midline of the tool. This line can be represented as the linear equation $y = mx + b$, where m is the slope and b is the intercept in the image plane. The state vector at the current time t is defined as $X_t = [m, b, m', b']^T$, where (m', b') denotes the first derivative of the slope intercept parameters. The KF tracking framework is composed of time update (prediction) and measurement update (correction). For each frame, the location of the tool's midline is predicted from previous frames, and the system model we obtain is then modified according to the selected measurements. Figure 4.11 illustrates the flowchart of a single iteration in the KF.

In the predication phase, both the *a priori* estimated state vector $\hat{X}_t^-$ and *a priori* estimated error covariance P_t^- are provided from the previous time, $t-1$. The prediction equation is defined as

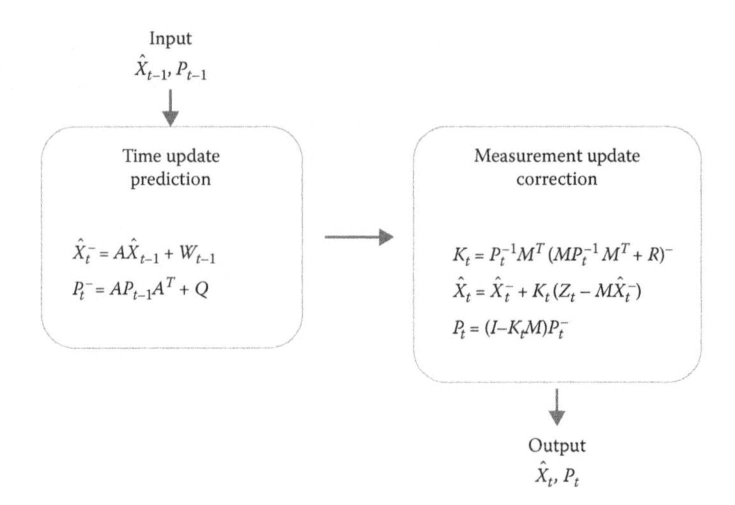

FIGURE 4.11 Information flow diagram of a single iteration in a standard KF implementation.

$$\hat{X}_t^- = A\hat{X}_{t-1} + W_{t-1} \Rightarrow \begin{bmatrix} m_t \\ b_t \\ m'_t \\ b'_t \end{bmatrix} = \begin{bmatrix} 1 & 0 & 1 & 0 \\ 0 & 1 & 0 & 1 \\ 0 & 0 & 1 & 0 \\ 0 & 0 & 0 & 1 \end{bmatrix} \begin{bmatrix} m_{t-1} \\ b_{t-1} \\ m'_{t-1} \\ b'_{t-1} \end{bmatrix} + W_{t-1}$$

$$P_t^- = AP_{t-1}A^T + Q$$

$$p(W_{t-1}) \sim N(0, Q) \tag{4.14}$$

where W_{t-1} is process noise with the noise covariance, and Q and A is the transition matrix.

Before we correct the *a priori* values $\hat{X}_t^-$ and P_t^-, we need to actually measure the process through image processing of the surgical scene to obtain Z_t, which is known as the measurement, in order to generate an improved posterior state estimate, $\hat{X}_t$. Corresponding to the state vector we defined, here, the real location of the tool's midline is used as the measurement $Z_t = [m, b]^T$, which can be expressed as

$$Z_t = MX_t + V_t \Rightarrow \begin{bmatrix} m_{\text{measure}\,t} \\ b_{\text{measure}\,t} \end{bmatrix} = \begin{bmatrix} 1 & 0 & 0 & 0 \\ 0 & 1 & 0 & 0 \end{bmatrix} \begin{bmatrix} m_t \\ b_t \\ m'_t \\ b'_t \end{bmatrix} + V_t$$

$$p(V_t) \sim N(0, R) \tag{4.15}$$

where V_t is the measurement noise with the noise covariance, and R and M is the measurement matrix. During 2-D feature recognition, the image after the Canny filter contains both useful and noisy information. The predicted midline is utilized to filter out unwanted edges according to the slope value of the edge candidates and their distances to the midline. After eliminating the disturbing line segments, we classify the remaining lines to be either the left or right edge and convert them into the slope intercept form. The posterior state $\hat{X}_t$ and error covariance P_t can be obtained from the following correction equations:

$$K_t = P_t^{-1} M^T \left(M P_t^{-1} M^T + R \right)^{-1}$$

$$\hat{X}_t = \hat{X}_t^- + K_t \left(Z_t - M \hat{X}_t^- \right)$$

$$P_t = \left(I - K_t M \right) P_t^- \tag{4.16}$$

where K refers to the gain matrix. At the end of each recursion, the corrected posterior values $\hat{X}_t$ and P_t turn out to be the input of the next time, $t+1$. The initialization of the KF framework requires the user's assistance to obtain the starting position for the tool's two edges. The initial midline at time $t+0$ is computed from the initial two edges. If the tracking is lost, the KF is reinitialized from the frame after the last one.

Besides the edges and the midline, the location of the tool tip is another significant feature. Since the surgical tool is usually made of a special material that is distinct from its surroundings, the tip position is probably among those points of dramatic change along the tool's midline. To avoid reflection spots and side effects, some noise reduction filters are implemented to reduce such effects. Generally, we start searching along the x direction (left to right). When the tool is almost vertical in the scene, we search then along the y direction.

After the initial prediction, through the proposed image processing, the location of the middle line is measured before the correction phase. The algorithm is the same as the edge detection algorithm in the initialization phase except that it takes advantage of the predicted state to filter out the edges that are unlikely to belong to the tool. Even if there are two tools or similar objects within the screen, the edges that belong to other objects won't be detected. The filter uses a simple comparison between the edge and the middle line. If the difference in the slopes between the measured edge and the predicated middle line is smaller than the threshold (i.e., $|m_{middleline} - m_{edge}| < \varepsilon$) and its edge point is close enough to the middle line $|d_{max}| < \varepsilon$, we assume this edge belongs to the tool. The slope of the middle line is shown as $m_{middleline}$, and m_{edge} is the slope of the edge; d_{max} is the maximum distance among the edge points and the middle line.

Modified Kalman Filter

In the previous implementation of the KF framework, 2-D feature recognition is defined using a somewhat consistent background and the gray scale of the image. In some cases, the tracking may be lost when more complex scenes are present. Generally, the background in surgical cases contains objects such as organs, tissue, and vessels. Considering this unique feature of the scene, some preprocessing procedures are required to eliminate noise from the background and meanwhile highlight useful feature structures such as edges. Instead of converting the RGB image into gray scale, we split the original (Figure 4.12a) into three single images (Figure 4.12b–d), where each of them contains information from only one color channel (red, green, or blue). By comparing the three single-channel images, we find details in the background become blurred in the red-channel image (d), so the following processing steps are

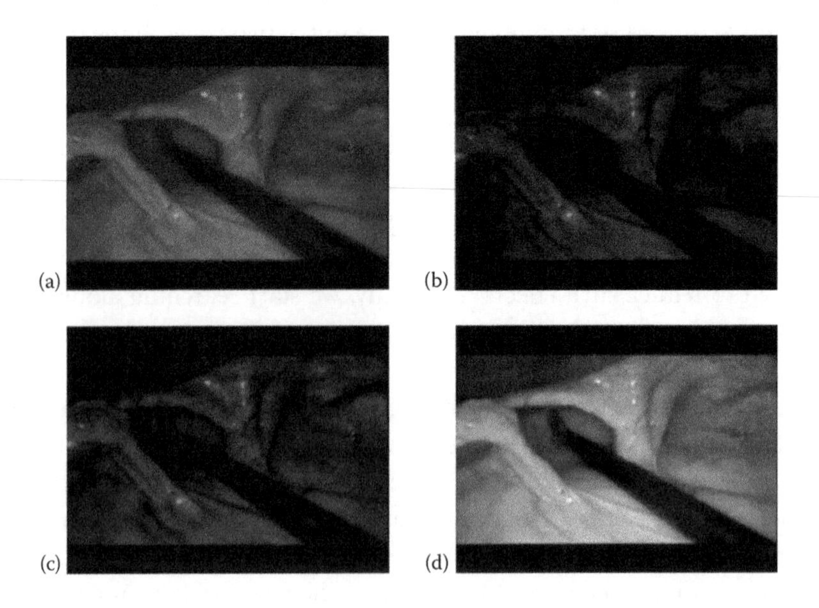

FIGURE 4.12 Example of an input image from the surgical scene: (a) the input image; (b) the blue-channel image; (c) the green-channel image; (d) the red-channel image.

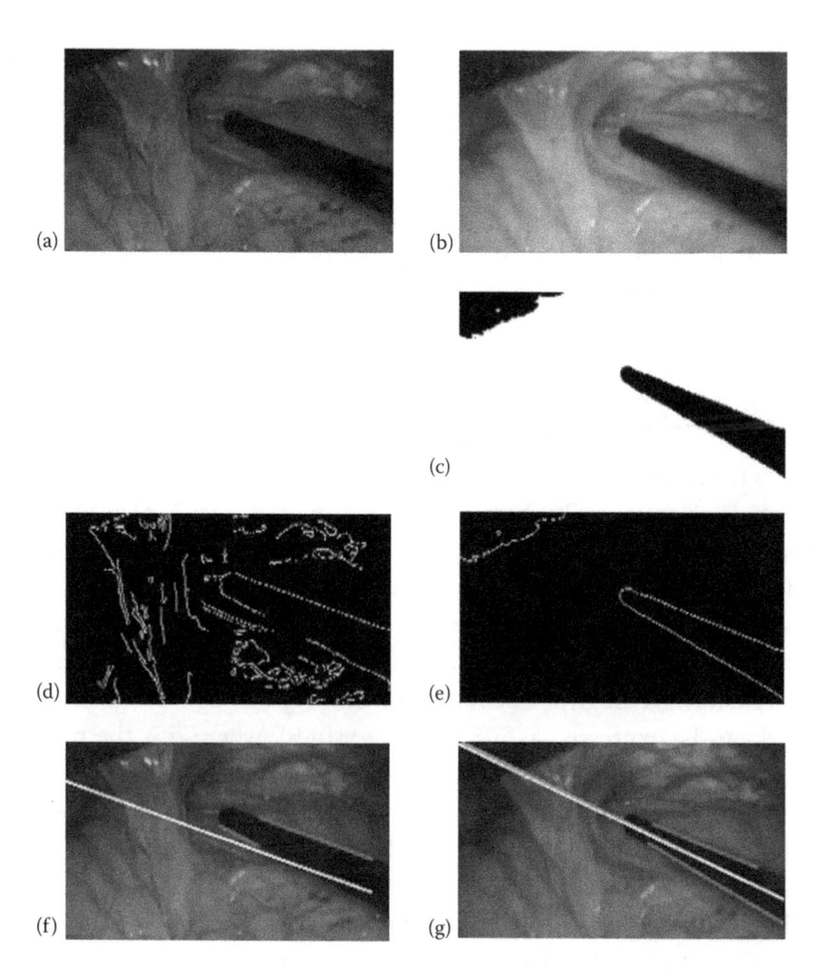

FIGURE 4.13 Comparison of the tracking performance between the original and modified KF method. The first column is for the original KF and the second column is for modified KF. (a) The gray scale image; (b) the red-channel image; (c) the image after binarization; (d–e) the Canny images for the original and modified KF, respectively. The tracking results can be seen in (f) and (g).

implemented. Before we use the Canny detector, a binary filter is applied on the red-channel image to highlight the tool since the colors of surgical tools are generally different from background images (e.g., dark black or gray-colored material). By adding the color split and binarization step, we have more reliably detected edges, which increases the accuracy of tracking. A comparison of the tracking results with and without modification is shown in Figure 4.13. The white line is the corrected midline of the surgical tool and the green line is the predicted midline. It can be seen that the modified KF method is more robust with respect to noise from the background.

Extended Kalman Filter

The standard KF tracking algorithm performs well in most cases when the movements of the surgical tool have nominal configuration and speed in both *in vitro* and *in vivo* settings. But this tracking framework has some limitations that are associated with the inclination angle of the surgical tool with respect to the endoscope axis. For example, due to the position of the incision point, the orientation of the tool may be very close to the vertical direction in the image plane. In this case, the magnitudes of both the slope and the intercept the of tool's midline tend to be infinite in vertical orientation. In these cases, the proposed tracking based on the standard KF needs to be enhanced in order to deal with these singular configurations. One possible solution is to redefine the description of the lines using polar parameters ρ and θ with respect to the image frame. This polar representation, defined in Figure 4.14, is from the Hough line transform (Hough 1962). Each line passing through the given point $P(x, y)$ can be expressed as $\rho = x\cos(\theta) + y\sin(\theta)$, where ρ is the perpendicular distance of the line to the origin and θ is the angle between the line and the reference axis. Since the representation of the line is now nonlinear, an extended Kalman filter (EKF) (Zarchan and Musoff 2009) is required in the new tracking framework. This type of nonlinear KF model is widely used in various fields such as unmanned aerial vehicle navigation (Rigatos 2012) and lane marking detection (Voisin et al. 2005; Borkar et al. 2009). Also, for detecting the edges of moving objects, a

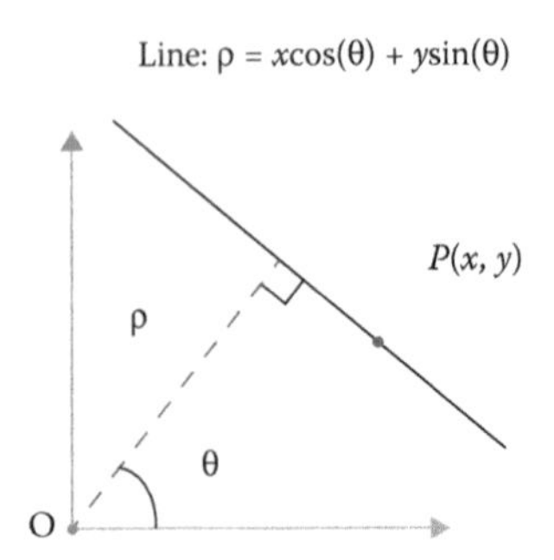

FIGURE 4.14 Polar representation of a line defined in Hough space.

combined tracking method using the KF and the Hough transform is proposed (Mills et al. 2003).

In the previous description of the standard KF method, the state vector is created from the midline of the surgical tool as $X_t = [m, b, m', b']^T$. For the EKF, the two edges of the surgical tool are selected for tracking purposes as opposed to the midline of the tool. Generally, the motion of the tool in the image plane can be decomposed into translation and rotation. Based on this decomposition, the following state vector is defined:

$$X_t = [x, y, u, v, w, \theta_1, \rho_1, \theta_2, \rho_2]^T \tag{4.17}$$

where (x, y) are the coordinates of the center of rotation, representing the motion of the tool. The translational velocities along the x and y axes are labeled as u and v, while w is the angular (rotational) velocity. In addition, (ρ_i, θ_i) $(i = 1, 2)$ are the representations of the line parameters of two edges of the tool. To simplify the computation, we assume both translation and rotation have a constant speed.

For example, for the current time (frame) t, the rotational center has been translated from (x_{t-1}, y_{t-1}) to (x_t, y_t) at speed (u_{t-1}, v_{t-1}). Hence, the state vector at time t can be defined as

$$\hat{X}_t^- = \begin{bmatrix} x_t \\ y_t \\ u_t \\ v_t \\ w_t \\ \theta_{1t} \\ \rho_{1t} \\ \theta_{2t} \\ \rho_{2t} \end{bmatrix} = \begin{bmatrix} x_{t-1} + u_{t-1} \\ y_{t-1} + v_{t-1} \\ u_{t-1} \\ v_{t-1} \\ w_{t-1} \\ \theta_{1(t-1)} + w_{t-1} \\ r_1(k-1) \\ \theta_{2(t-1)} + w_{t-1} \\ r_2(k-1) \end{bmatrix} = f\left(\hat{X}_{t-1}\right) \tag{4.18}$$

with

$$\begin{aligned} r_i(t-1) = {} & \rho_{i(t-1)} - x_{t-1}\cos\left(\theta_{i(t-1)}\right) - y_{t-1}\sin\left(\theta_{i(t-1)}\right) + x_t\cos\left(\theta_{it}\right) \\ & + y_t\sin\left(\theta_{it}\right), \quad i = 1,2 \end{aligned}$$

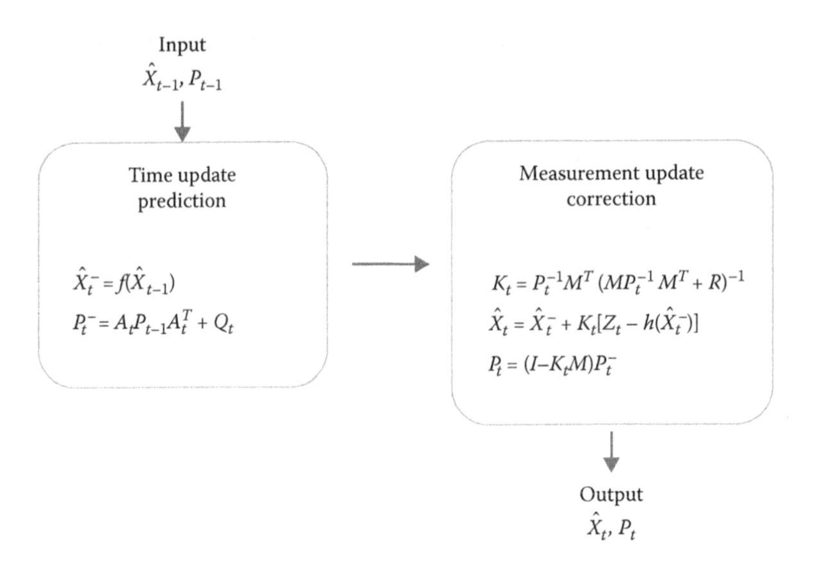

FIGURE 4.15 Flow diagram for a single iteration of the EKF.

The measurement for the EKF is the observed location of two edges, which is

$$Z_t = \left[\theta_{1t\ \text{real}}, \rho_{1t\ \text{real}}, \theta_{2t\ \text{real}}, \rho_{2t\ \text{real}}\right]^T = h(X_t) \tag{4.19}$$

Figure 4.15 demonstrates the information flow for a single iteration in the EKF. The transition matrix A in the prediction stage is defined as

$$A_{[i,j]} = \frac{\partial f_{[i]}}{\partial X_{[j]}}(\hat{X}_t) \Rightarrow A = \begin{bmatrix} 1 & 0 & 1 & 0 & 0 & 0 & 0 & 0 & 0 \\ 0 & 1 & 0 & 1 & 0 & 0 & 0 & 0 & 0 \\ 0 & 0 & 1 & 0 & 0 & 0 & 0 & 0 & 0 \\ 0 & 0 & 0 & 1 & 0 & 0 & 0 & 0 & 0 \\ 0 & 0 & 0 & 0 & 1 & 0 & 0 & 0 & 0 \\ 0 & 0 & 0 & 0 & 1 & 1 & 0 & 0 & 0 \\ \frac{\partial \rho_1}{\partial x} & \frac{\partial \rho_1}{\partial y} & \frac{\partial \rho_1}{\partial u} & \frac{\partial \rho_1}{\partial v} & \frac{\partial \rho_1}{\partial w} & \frac{\partial \rho_1}{\partial \theta_1} & 1 & 0 & 0 \\ 0 & 0 & 0 & 0 & 1 & 0 & 0 & 1 & 0 \\ \frac{\partial \rho_2}{\partial x} & \frac{\partial \rho_2}{\partial y} & \frac{\partial \rho_2}{\partial u} & \frac{\partial \rho_2}{\partial v} & \frac{\partial \rho_2}{\partial w} & 0 & 0 & \frac{\partial \rho_2}{\partial \theta_2} & 1 \end{bmatrix} \tag{4.20}$$

For the correction period, the measurement matrix M takes the form of

$$M_{[m,j]} = \frac{\partial h_{[m]}}{\partial X_{[j]}}(\hat{X}^{-})_t \Rightarrow M = \begin{bmatrix} 0 & 0 & 0 & 0 & 0 & 1 & 0 & 0 & 0 \\ 0 & 0 & 0 & 0 & 0 & 0 & 1 & 0 & 0 \\ 0 & 0 & 0 & 0 & 0 & 0 & 0 & 1 & 0 \\ 0 & 0 & 0 & 0 & 0 & 0 & 0 & 0 & 1 \end{bmatrix} \tag{4.21}$$

According to Hough (1962) line transform theory, given an arbitrary point $P(x, y)$ in the Cartesian image space, we can draw a corresponding curve (i.e., sinusoids) in the Hough space that indicates all the possible lines in the image space passing through the point P. For those points that are collinear in the image plane, their corresponding curves in the Hough space will intersect at a common point (θ, ρ). These intersections are called peaks. Generally, the Hough space is stored using a matrix, whose element value indicates the number of curves passing through the point (θ, ρ). Peaks are expressed as local maxima in this matrix that correspond to straight lines in the image plane.

The visual tracking of a surgical tool is conducted inside a body cavity, where the rigid tool is surrounded by soft organs and tissue. Here it is assumed that the surgical tool has the most salient line structure, which also implies that the two maximum peaks also correspond to two edges of the tool. For the time instance t, the estimated peak position from the previous time $t-1$ is used to limit the search area for the real location of the edges. For example, Figure 4.16 shows part of the Hough transform matrix (Zhou and Payandeh 2014). The search area for finding peaks in values is restrained inside the red rectangle, which is obtained based on the estimated state vector from time $t-1$. In Figure 4.16, red circles indicate the two maximum peaks that were found inside this area. The measure Z_t derives from these two peaks and is used to correct the next predicted peak position for time t.

Adaptive Gaussian Mixture Model (AGGM)

Another approach for detecting a moving object in an image sequence is based on background subtraction. The adaptive Gaussian mixture model (AGMM) is an approach that has applications in a number of visual tracking problems. The basic idea of the AGMM is to set up a background model that can be used to distinguish the foreground object from the background environment. By calculating a reference image and subtracting each new

θ →

ρ ↓

34	9	3	4	4	4	4	5	7	4	3	6
11	22	9	4	5	4	4	5	4	5	7	4
4	28	17	3	4	4	7	4	6	4	3	6
11	6	25	8	4	4	5	2	5	3	6	4
23	9	20	31	1	4	4	4	5	6	5	4
10	25	13	14	12	3	4	6	3	4	4	7
10	16	23	26	31	4	3	6	5	5	4	2
12	10	16	30	23	20	5	5	4	6	3	5
6	6	14	16	44	34	11	4	5	5	6	5
12	7	2	5	15	43	33	6	5	4	4	4
23	3	4	6	3	23	35	42	11	4	6	6
20	21	6	3	3	3	25	21	34	17	5	3
11	26	11	5	6	3	17	22	23	21	21	8
16	21	19	11	4	4	4	21	20	20	18	18
15	17	36	17	6	4	4	16	7	25	12	16
7	14	28	29	23	6	3	2	23	15	24	11
3	4	9	39	31	21	3	4	15	6	18	17
2	2	2	8	30	44	20	3	4	18	9	22
2	3	2	5	10	14	51	21	10	18	7	12
2	2	2	2	7	14	6	40	17	15	19	8
2	2	2	1	6	4	19	17	31	15	28	16
2	1	2	1	2	9	5	7	16	24	19	18
1	2	0	2	2	6	2	17	10	18	16	26
1	2	3	2	2	3	9	2	16	6	20	26
1	1	2	2	2	3	6	2	10	15	9	19
0	1	2	2	2	1	6	7	2	16	6	11
1	1	2	2	2	2	2	7	2	7	16	5
1	1	0	2	1	2	2	7	5	1	15	8
1	1	1	2	2	2	2	4	7	3	7	17
1	1	1	1	2	2	2	1	6	3	2	13

FIGURE 4.16 Searching for the peak values in the Hough space.

frame from this reference image, we can highlight the region of the moving object.

A multicolor background model was originally developed per pixel to solve dynamic object detection, which also set the basis for the development of the AGMM (Grimson et al. 1998) (Appendix III). This method was later improved by introducing a shadow detection scheme, which offers a more robust performance with respect to slight changes in the environment (Kaewtrakulpong and Bowden 2002). Other developments included the use of recursive equations to continuously update the parameters and adjust the number of components associated with each pixel.

In the implementation of the AGMM, the pixel values in the scene background are modeled using a mixture of adaptive Gaussian components. Pixels that do not match with the background Gaussian components are classified as foreground pixels. Given an arbitrary pixel value x_t, the ith Gaussian density function at time t can be written as $\eta(x_t, \mu_{i,t}, \sigma_{i,t}^2)$ with a mean value $\mu_{i,t}$ and a standard deviation $\sigma_{i,t}$. The probability of a particular pixel p_0 having value x_t is defined as

$$P(x_t) = \sum_{i=1}^{k} w_{i,t}\eta\left(x_t, \mu_{i,t}, \sigma_{i,t}^2\right)$$

where $w_{i,t}$ is the weight for the ith Gaussian component and k is the number of components. In general, the background scene is not absolutely fixed but has some slight changes. For example, as a related problem, the moving leaves on a tree can cause a slight change in the background even if the camera is placed at a fixed location. Changing of the illuminant associated with the environment can be another contributing factor to changes in the background image. To cope with these types of problems, an adaptive background model is proposed. Here, the weights of each of the Gaussian components are updated as a function of the current time t. To allow a foreground object to become part of the background later, the Gaussian distribution with the lowest weight is replaced with a new Gaussian function. This new Gaussian component is given a low normalized weight that will be used at time $t+1$. Meanwhile, the mean and variance of the other remaining Gaussian components for time $t+1$ are also updated.

In general, the AGMM method is able to return the foreground object region but it contains some shadow noise. To deal with this problem, a shadow elimination step is added to the output of the AGMM. Furthermore, to reduce the remaining noise, morphological operations such as opening and closing are also applied to the shadow-detected image. After these postprocessing steps, the contour of the moving surgical tool is extracted frame by frame. An information flow diagram for the AGMM tracking framework is shown in Figure 4.17. Some examples of the intermediate steps associated with this approach are shown in Figure 4.18.

SURGICAL TOOL TIP EXTRACTION

Once the two edges have been extracted, it remains to determine the relative position of the surgical tool tip. In order to localize the tip, the 1-D profile of the image along the middle line for each tool is computed. By performing 1-D edge detection along the middle line of the image profile,

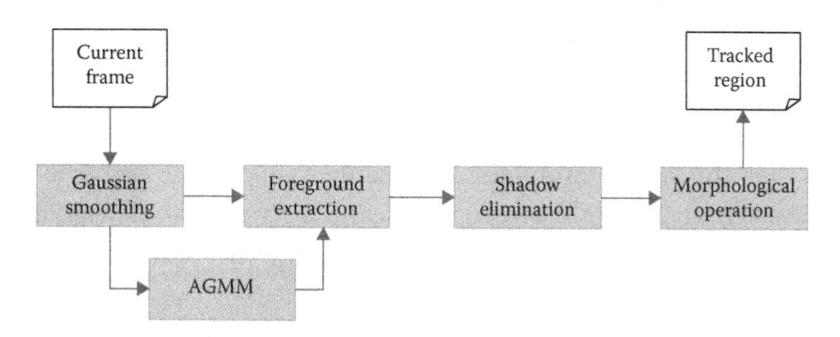

FIGURE 4.17 Flow diagram of AGMM implementation in surgical tool tracking.

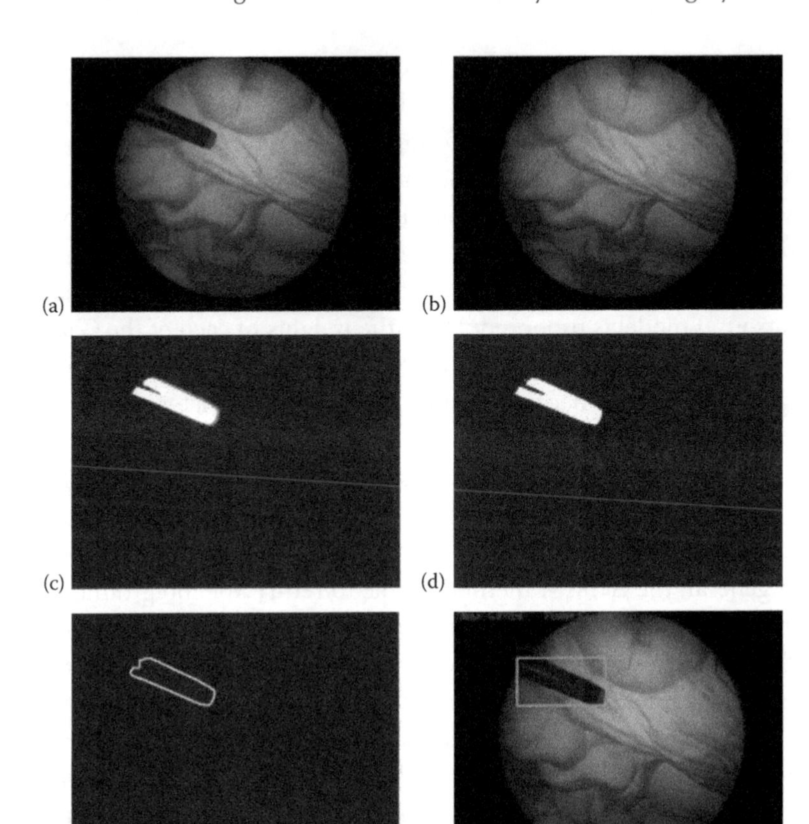

FIGURE 4.18 Intermediate steps for the AGMM approach: (a) the input image; (b) the background image; (c) the extracted foreground object; (d) after shadow elimination; (e) the contour of the tool extracted after morphological operation; (f) the region containing the moving tool.

the tip location, which corresponds to the largest change of the pixel values, can be extracted.

In general, the tip is localized where there exists a sudden change of intensity, since there exists a noticeable pixel contrast between the tool and its background. However, when the light changes and reflection occurs on the tool, the algorithm might mistakenly interpret the tip to be at the reflection spot instead of the expected location. To prevent such situations, which occur quite often in real surgical operations, various filters have been implemented.

There are three filters added in order to minimize the effect of such noise. The first one is to extract the hue, saturation, and value (HSV) of the

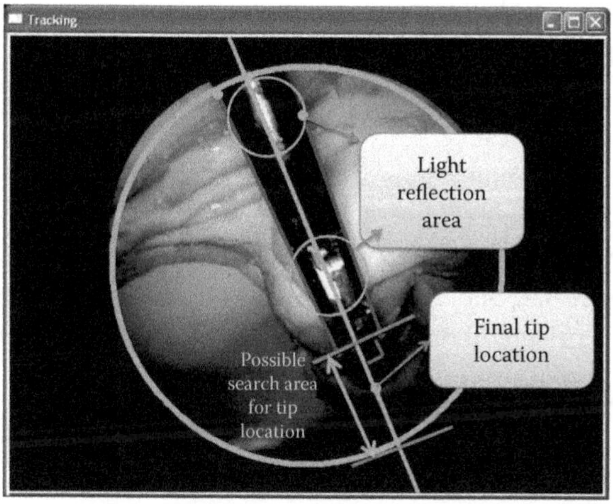

FIGURE 4.19 Tip extraction search area after applying filters.

pixel; when the value is above a certain threshold, which implies that the location has a high probability of being a source of light reflection, the algorithm stores this possible location and searches again for the next possible pixel location on the middle line. As shown in Figure 4.19, the *light reflection area* will be avoided by applying this filter. The second filter is used to decide whether the extracted possible tip location is valid given the orientation of the edges with respect to the endoscope. In other words, the tip is always along the side where the geometric representation of the edges can intersect. If the detected tip location is within the location of the edges or located on the wrong side of the intersection point, it is discarded. Finally, the last filter is designed to ensure that the tip location is not located at the border of the endoscopic image, since there exists a sharp intensity between the background and the circle border of the endoscopic images. Figure 4.19 shows an arrow indicating the *possible search area* that can be affected when applying the last two filters. The green circle is the border of the endoscopic image, and the possible search area starts from the end point of the edges (whichever is farthest away along the middle line) and ends at the border. By applying the second and third filter, the possible search area is minimized to be within an edge point and the border. In this way, it is possible to reduce noise and other effects in a light-variant environment.

In this algorithm, to search for the tip location, we can search along the horizontal direction (i.e., the x direction), which is to calculate the intensity difference from the leftmost pixel to the rightmost. However, when the tool is almost vertical in the scene, this approach is very inaccurate since the searchable area for the tip location is suddenly very small; in which case, a vertical (y) search is applied. In order to enhance the algorithm, two separate conditions are defined as a function slope or orientation of the surgical tool (Figure 4.20). As a result and regardless of how the tool is oriented, the tip localizer is always able to search for the valid tip location. Figure 4.21 shows two screenshots from the image frames. One of the tools is oriented horizontally, the other is vertically inserted; both have been detected successfully.

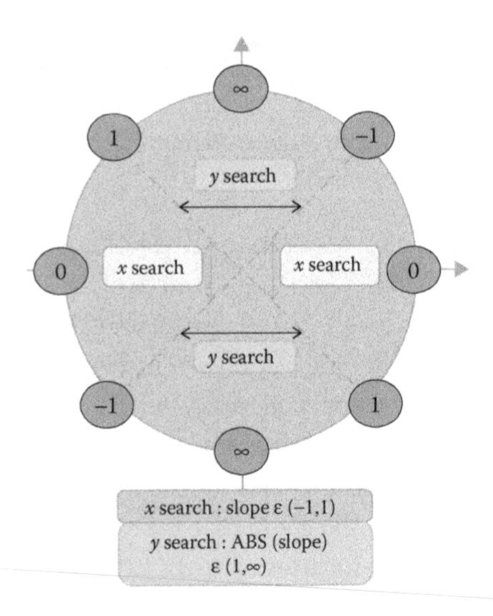

FIGURE 4.20 Schematic of the tool tip extraction strategy.

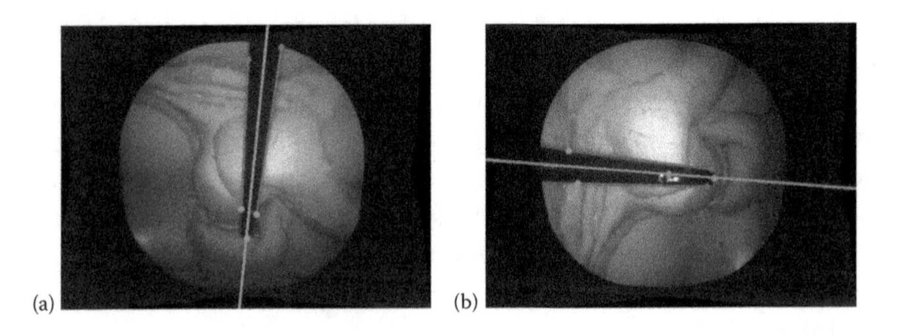

FIGURE 4.21 Examples of surgical tool tip tracking results: (a) tip search in the x direction; (b) tip search in the y direction.

Two-Dimensional Tracking of Multiple Tools

Tracking multiple surgical tools can be an important aspect of developing an advanced SCI. Being able to track two surgical tools is analogous to tracking the two hands of the surgeon. By manipulating the two tools, the surgeon is able to grab, rotate, and translate an overlaid image/3-D object. A suitable tracking system has to be adopted in order to support tracking of multiple tools. For example, a method for tracking the movements of two surgical tools using blob analysis of different colors was proposed by Salajegheh (2008). However, the approach is not robust when the tip is occluded. Additionally, since it lacks the ability to reconstruct the orientation of the tool, it cannot provide spatial information regarding the surgical tool. The MHI approach (discussed previously) can track multiple tools, but when the tools are crossing each other's paths, the tracking information can be lost.

The proposed algorithm supports the tracking of multiple surgical tools based on the KF. The edge that doesn't belong to the tool is filtered during image processing, and as a result, multiple tracking can be applied individually. To support multiple-tool tracking, a second KF is added that is initialized with predefined values for m and b combined with the second tool tip extraction. Figure 4.22a shows the initialization procedure by placing the tool around the two green lines. The two lines ($E_1(m_1, b_1)$, $E_2(m_2, b_2)$) are initialized as (−1.0, 550.0) and (1.0, −50.0). Through the second tool tip extraction, the intersecting region between the two middle

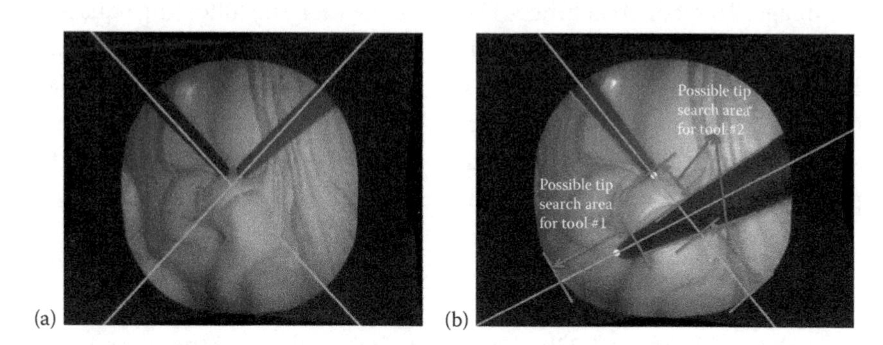

FIGURE 4.22 Two modifications of the tracking algorithm to adapt multiple tracking. (a) The initialization is achieved by placing the tool around the two lines. The lines ($E_1[m_1, b_1]$) and ($E_2[m_2, b_2]$) are initialized as (−1.0, 550.0) and (1.0, −50.0). (b) The tip search area is modified so that the area between one tool's middle line intersecting with another tool's two edges is removed. The two sided arrow regions represent the valid search area for each of the tools.

lines of the tools is removed (as shown in Figure 4.22b) where the intensity changes occur.

SURGICAL TOOL TRACKING IN 3-D

This section proposes an approach for obtaining depth and relative positional information between instruments. The proposed image analysis extracts information from the projective geometry of the surgical setting in the image to determine the position of the surgical tools. The cylindrical geometry of the instruments and their projective contours in the image are utilized to estimate the orientations of the surgical tools and their spatial positions.

Three-Dimensional Pose Estimation Using Surgical Tool Tip and Edges

This section utilizes the information obtained from the previous analysis and results (2-D edges and the associated surgical tool tip) to reconstruct the 3-D pose of the tool with respect to the endoscope. It takes advantage of the geometrical properties of the rigid cylindrical instrument to calculate the 3-D tip location as well as the orientation (or 3-D vector) of the tool axis. Other prior knowledge is that the camera is fully calibrated and the physical diameter ($d_{physical}$) of the tool is given.

In the previous chapter, it was noted that due to the projective geometry of the endoscopic scene, the cylindrical tool is visualized as a trapezoid in the image. To reconstruct the 3-D pose of the tool, the following equations are derived using projective geometry (Cano et al. 2006) (Figure 4.23). $E1$ and $E2$ are two edges of the surgical tool projected onto the image plane. T is the tip of the tool in the 2-D image, with the 3-D coordinate as P. The camera center is denoted as C, while θ is the angle between the physical tool with respect to the image plane.

$$\vec{u}_{\Omega i} = \vec{u}_{Ei} \times \vec{u}_{CEi}, \quad i-1,2 \tag{4.22}$$

As shown in Figure 4.23b, the angle λ_N between one of the symmetrical planes to the CN vector can be expressed by addition of the normal vector of ($u_{\Omega 1}$ and $u_{\Omega 2}$):

$$\tan\lambda_N = \frac{\left|\vec{u}_{\Omega 1} + \vec{u}_{\Omega 2}\right|}{\left|\vec{u}_{\Omega 1} - \vec{u}_{\Omega 2}\right|} \tag{4.23}$$

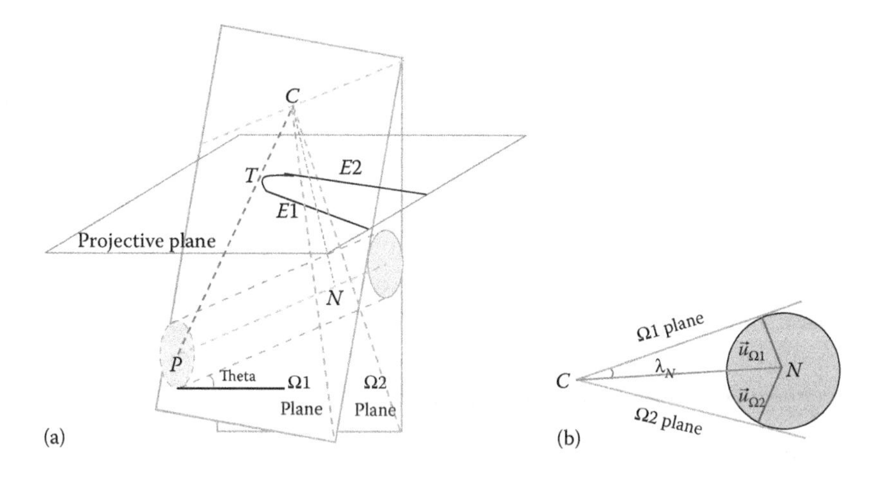

FIGURE 4.23 (a) 3-D projective model; (b) the transverse section of the projective model. Two tangential planes Ω1 and Ω2 that include one of the edges on the tool and the camera vector to the edge are defined. The normal vector $(\vec{u}_{\Omega 1}, \vec{u}_{\Omega 2})$ to each tangential plane is obtained through the cross product of the edges $(\vec{u}_{E1}, \vec{u}_{E2})$ and the camera $(\vec{u}_{CE1}, \vec{u}_{CE2})$ to the edge.

To determine the length of the *CN* vector (Figure 4.23b)—namely, the distance from the camera to the tool axis—we can apply the prior knowledge of the tool radius as

$$\left|CN\right| = \frac{d_{\text{physical}} . 0.5}{\sin \lambda_N} \tag{4.24}$$

The orientation of the *CN* vector can be simply derived as

$$\vec{u}_{CN} = \left|CN\right| \cdot \frac{\vec{u}_{\Omega 1} + \vec{u}_{\Omega 2}}{\left|\vec{u}_{\Omega 1} + \vec{u}_{\Omega 2}\right|} \tag{4.25}$$

Finally, the *CP* vector is determined as

$$\overrightarrow{CP} = \frac{\left|CN\right| \cdot \vec{u}_{CT}}{\vec{u}_{CT} \cdot \vec{u}_{CN}} \tag{4.26}$$

Note that *P* can be any point on the tool—in this case, the tip of the tool. Therefore, $\overrightarrow{CP}$ represents the vector from the camera origin *C* to the tip, meaning that the 3-D location of the tool is extracted. Moreover, the vector $\overrightarrow{NP}$ representing the orientation of the tool can be calculated as

$$\overrightarrow{NP} = -\overrightarrow{CN} + \overrightarrow{CP} \tag{4.27}$$

When $\overrightarrow{NP}$ is known, any other point of the tool can be obtained by knowing the physical distance between P and the desired point. Figure 4.24 shows the 2-D edge and tip information along with the reconstructed 3-D pose rendered by OpenGL. Up to this point, all the information needed has been extracted. The only degree of freedom we cannot detect is the rotation of the instrument around its axis (roll). Other than this, the left–right and forward–backward rotations of the instrument around the incision point (yaw and pitch) can be extracted.

EXPERIMENTAL STUDIES

This section presents the 2-D and 3-D results of the feature-based algorithm. Based on the previous section, the 2-D algorithm takes advantage of Kalman filtering to filter the invalid edges. The 3-D algorithm uses the detected edges and tip to reconstruct the tool position and orientation. In addition, the multiple-tool tracking result is also presented in order to demonstrate the feasibility of this approach.

Single-Tool Tracking

This subsection presents the tracking results for the single tool in the scene. The KF implementation allows the correct recognition of edges even though there are similar objects in the scene (Figure 4.25a,b). When the tool is partially occluded by another surgical tool (Figure 4.25c), the algorithm is able to recover the edges. Another advantage of the proposed tracking algorithm is that it can handle a certain level of light reflection. This is because the proposed surgical tool tip detection is independent

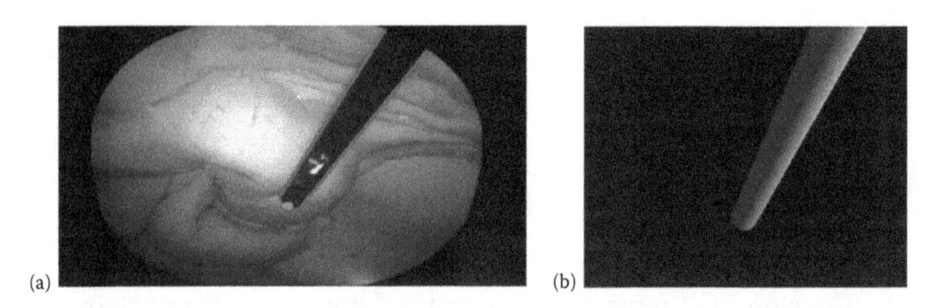

FIGURE 4.24 (a) Image with detected 2-D edges and tip; (b) reconstructed tool rendered in OpenGL.

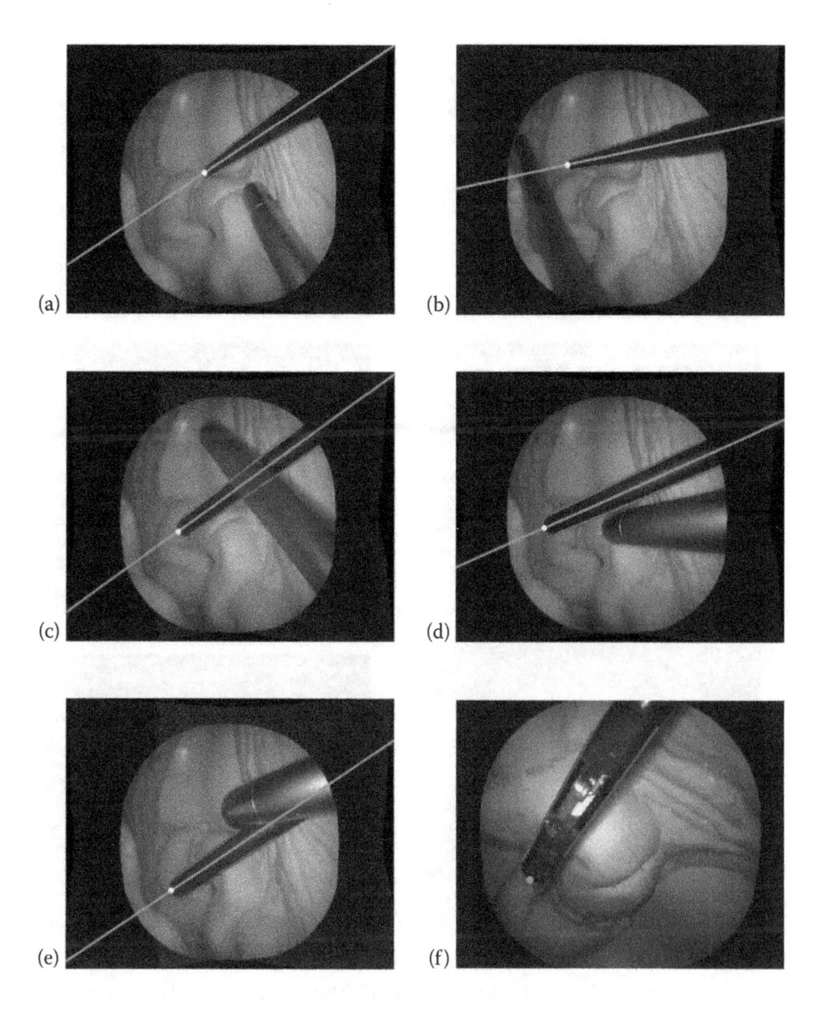

FIGURE 4.25 Screenshots of the successful tracking results: (a–b) The current algorithm can handle similar objects in the scene by implementing Kalman filtering. (c) The edges belonging to the tool can be recovered even though part of the tool is being occluded. (d–e) The edge detection can handle two similar tools with included angles larger than 20°–30°. (f) The current tip extraction module can handle some amount of light reflection caused by special material.

of the presence of light reflection, which allows successful recognition of the tip. Figure 4.25f shows the algorithm has a robust performance where there is the presence of a bright light on the metal part of the tool.

The performance of the tracking algorithm is evaluated in handling the partial occlusion of and similarities between objects and the effect of light reflection. In low-intensity light, the surgical tool cannot be recognized

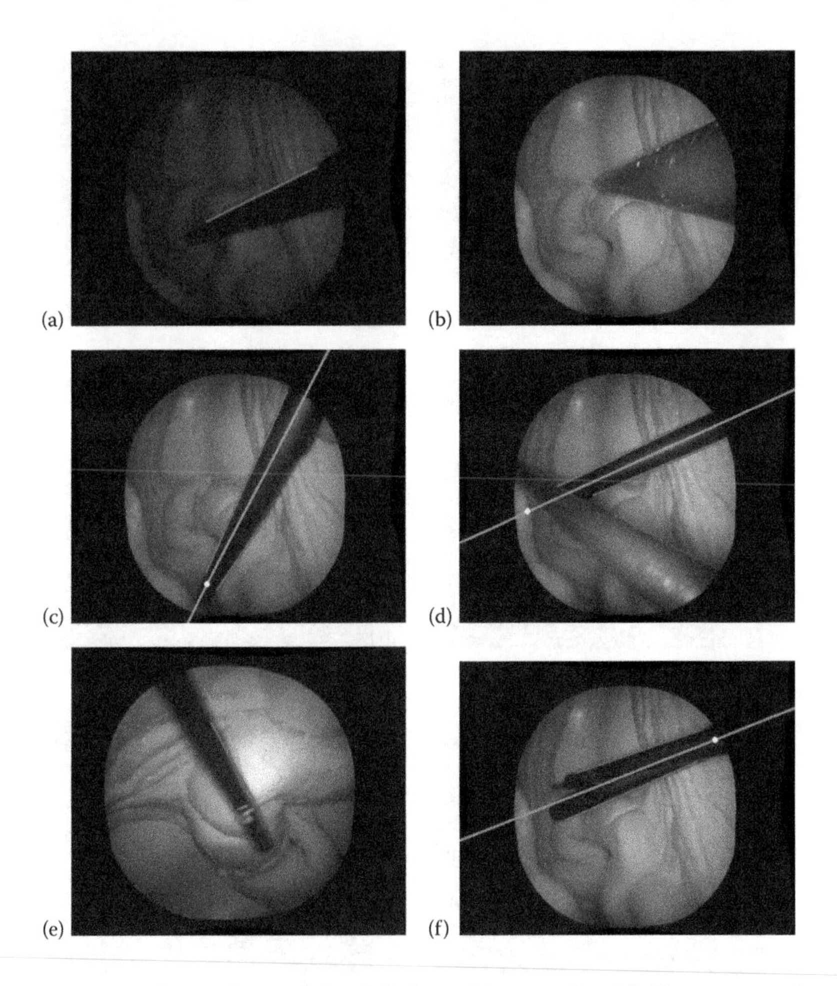

FIGURE 4.26 Screenshots of the failed tracking results: (a) The current algorithm fails to detect edges when the light is weak (under 30% of the maximum illumination setting in this case). (b) The shadow blurs the image, causing misdetection of the edge. (c) The tip extraction module fails to detect the correct tip due to lower contrast of the tip with respect to the background. (d) When the tip is occluded, the detection fails. (e) The current algorithm cannot handle the fast motion of the tool. (f) The edge detection cannot handle two similar tools with included angle less than 20°–30°.

properly since there is not enough contrast with respect to the background. Moreover, the shadow of the surgical tools will blur the sharp edge of the tool, making the edge detection fail, as shown in Figure 4.26a,c. Partial occlusion occurs occasionally in real surgical circumstances, such as when a tool is occluded by organs and tissues. There are successful cases of handling the occlusion. However, when the tool tip is being occluded, the algorithm performs poorly, though it can still anticipate the location of the surgical tool tip (Figure 4.26d).

When the tool moves fast enough (e.g., ≥8 cm/s), the movement causes blurs in the images; thus, the algorithm fails to detect the edges (as shown in Figure 4.26e). In general, however, the algorithm is robust enough to capture the images when they move moderately fast.

The detection also fails when a similar object approaches the tracking target and is oriented the same or the opposite way, which includes angles less than 20°–30°. However, this would not happen in real surgery, where the tools are generally farther apart, separated by incision points. Figure 4.25d,e are two successful tracking results with two objects having similar inclination angles with respect to the axis of the endoscope. However, when the two tools have overlapping inclination angles (Figure 4.26f), the tracking is lost. The algorithm mistakenly recognizes the edge belonging to another tool, causing incorrect edge and tip extraction.

In order to test the robustness and performance of the algorithm, disturbances resulting from tissue occlusion, the physical movement of the tool, and light variance are taken into consideration in the following experiments. Results of the image analysis have been grouped with respect to the input factors (Table 4.1). In these experiments, it has been assumed that the tool tip is found correctly if the position error is not greater than twice the width of the tool and the tool's orientation is found within 20° of error range. The number of frames experimented is 50 frames per subtest tracking under the corresponding input environments.

The results show that the current algorithm can handle some amount of noise and can be adopted as a reliable tracking system given nominal conditions when the tool speed is 0–4 cm/s, the percentage of brightness is within 46%–100%, and no similar objects are present within the scene.

TABLE 4.1 Experimental Results of Current Featured-Based Tracking Algorithm with Different Input Factors

Input Factors	**Range**	**Rate of Success (%)**
Tool speed (cm/s)	(0–4)	82
	(4–8)	54
	(9–∞)	32
Rate of brightness (%)	(0–30)	22
	(30–45)	52
	(46–100)	89
Distraction from similar objects (%)	95	

Multiple-Tool Tracking

Figure 4.27 shows screenshots of the successful multiple-tool tracking results. The algorithm works well even though one tool is on top of the other. Though a part of the tool is occluded, the edge detection procedure is able to recover the edges based on the assumption that the tool is cylindrically shaped. However, the tip extraction fails if it is occluded or is located beneath or on top of the other surgical tool (as shown in Figure 4.28a). Another tracking challenge is when the tools have small inclination angles (Figure 4.28b).

For the *in vivo* experiments, 10 video streams of various endoscopic procedures are used for evaluating the tracking performance of the proposed methods (KF, EKF, and AGMM). Each video stream lasts for about 10 s and contains about 200–300 frames. The surgical instruments are used to perform various complex procedures involving occlusion,

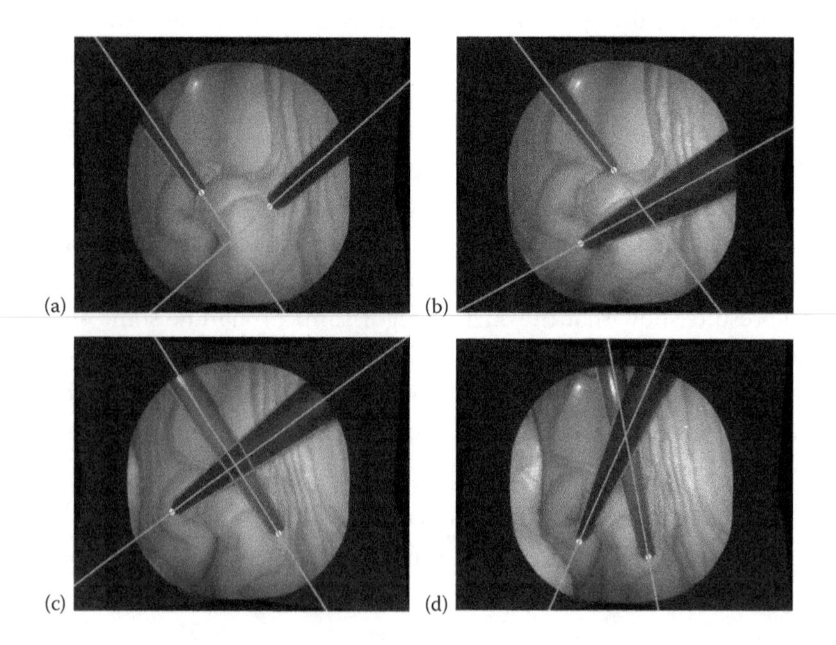

FIGURE 4.27 Multiple tracking results with successful cases. The long lines are the tools' middle lines, the shorter long segments are their edges, and the white spots are the detected tips. (a) The condition when two tools are separate to each other; (b) the condition when the tools' intersection point is on one of the tools' middle line; (c) the condition when two tools are crossing; (d) the condition when the tools' included angle is 30°.

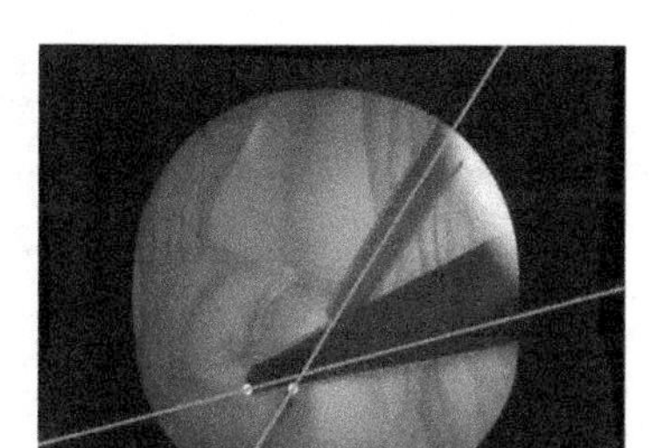

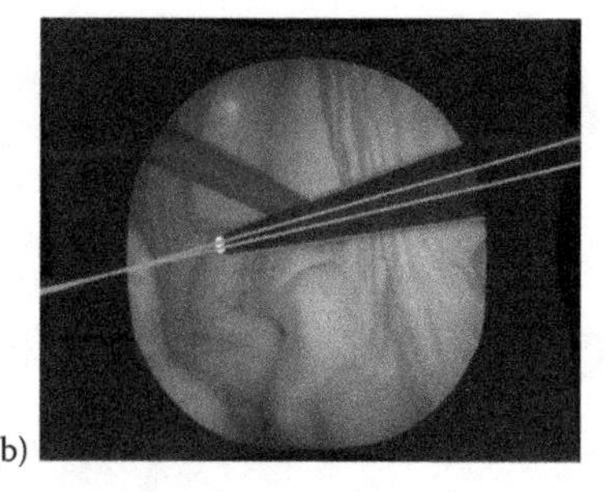

(a) (b)

FIGURE 4.28 Multiple tracking results with failed cases. The green lines are the tools' middle lines, the red are their edges, and the white spots are the detected tips. (a) The condition when one tool's tip is beneath another tool; (b) the condition when the tools have small inclination angles.

TABLE 4.2 Tracking Performance of KF, EKF, and AGMM Using Surgical Scenes

	Tracking Success Rate (frames/200 frames *100%)		
Method	**KF**	**EKF**	**AGMM**
Video no. 1	30%	48%	42%
Video no. 2	48%	33%	53%
Video no. 3	52%	Fail	38%
Video no. 4	Fail	50%	55%
Video no. 5	45%	31%	48%
Video no. 6	20%	18%	23%
Video no. 7	Fail	Fail	10%
Video no. 8	Fail	Fail	Fail
Video no. 9	Fail	Fail	Fail
Video no. 10	10%	Fail	12%

moving in and out of the camera's view, zooming in and out, and fast motion.

The tracking success rates that are tabulated in Table 4.2 are estimated from relatively stable cases. For videos no. 1, no. 2, no. 3, no. 5, and no. 6, the surface of the tool is dark and matt. For videos no. 4 and no. 7, the tool is made of a metallic material. Video no. 8 involves multiple-tool tasking. In video no. 9, the tool is moving at a relatively faster speed, and video no. 10 has a complex background. Figures 4.29 through 4.31 are examples of the tracking performance. In each figure, the first two rows are their successful tracking results, while failures are shown in the following two rows.

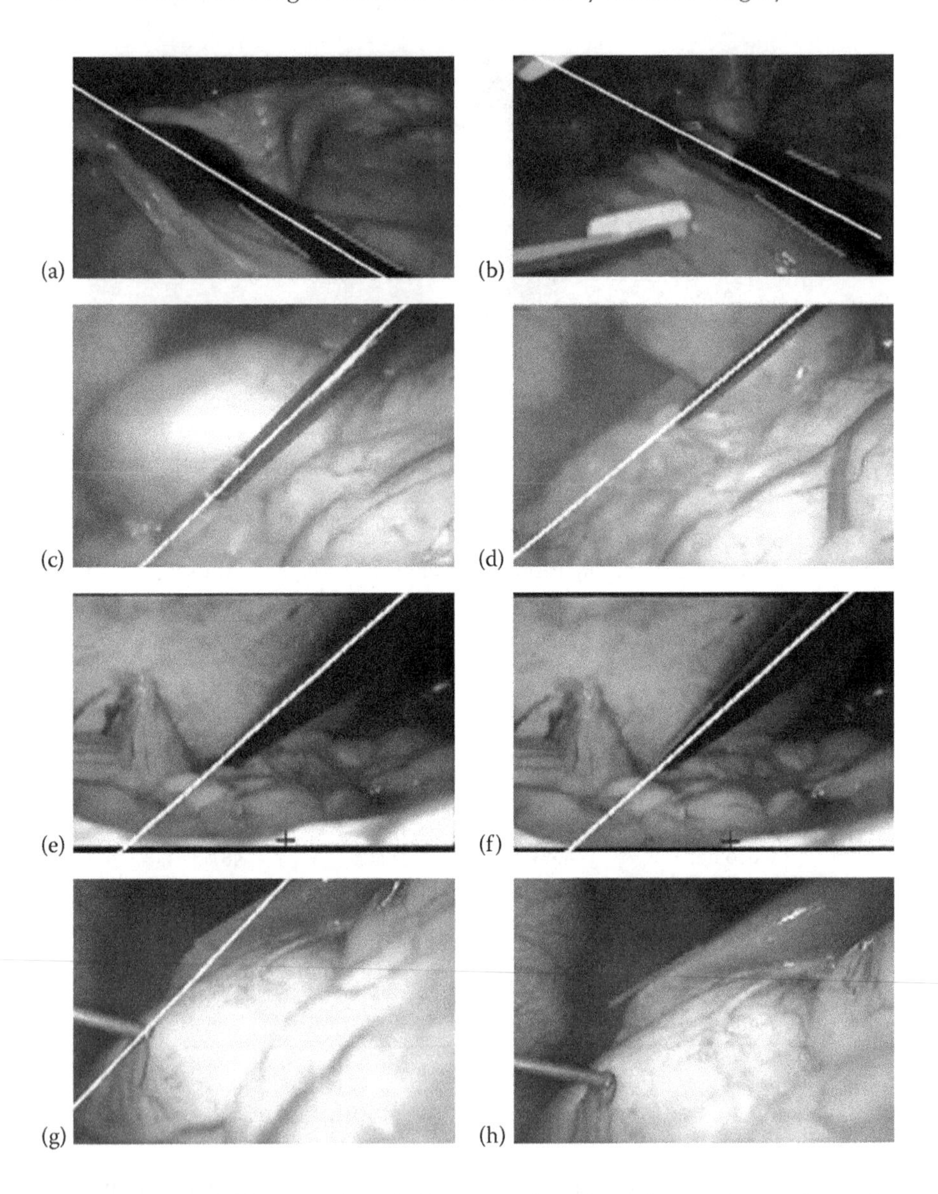

FIGURE 4.29 (a-h) Examples of KF surgical tool tracking using endoscopic video of the surgical scene.

THREE-DIMENSIONAL INTERACTIVE SURGICAL MOUSE

This section presents a preliminary 3-D interactive system based on the proposed tracking procedure using the markerless tracking framework. Here we propose a simple SCI for allowing the surgeon to access medical information and preoperative images during the surgery by using the

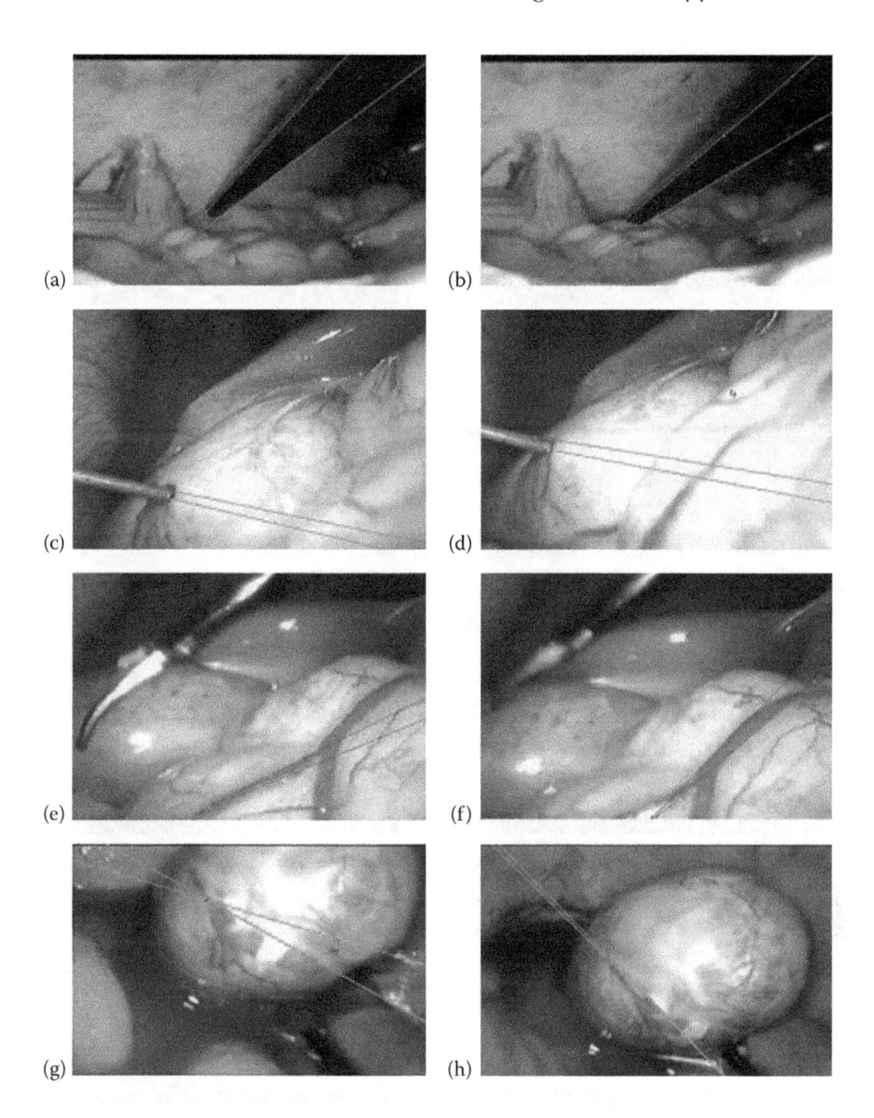

FIGURE 4.30 (a-h) Examples of EKF surgical tool tracking using endoscopic video of the surgical scene.

existing surgical tools operated by surgeons. As stated previously, our proposed system does not require any extra pieces of hardware and uses the existing imaging system to provide this novel SCI.

Instead of using stereoscopic head-tracked displays, we use a mono-camera and augmented reality (AR) to allow surgeons to interact with virtual reality. AR combines computer graphics with images of the real world. This can be accomplished through the use of video mixing, 3-D

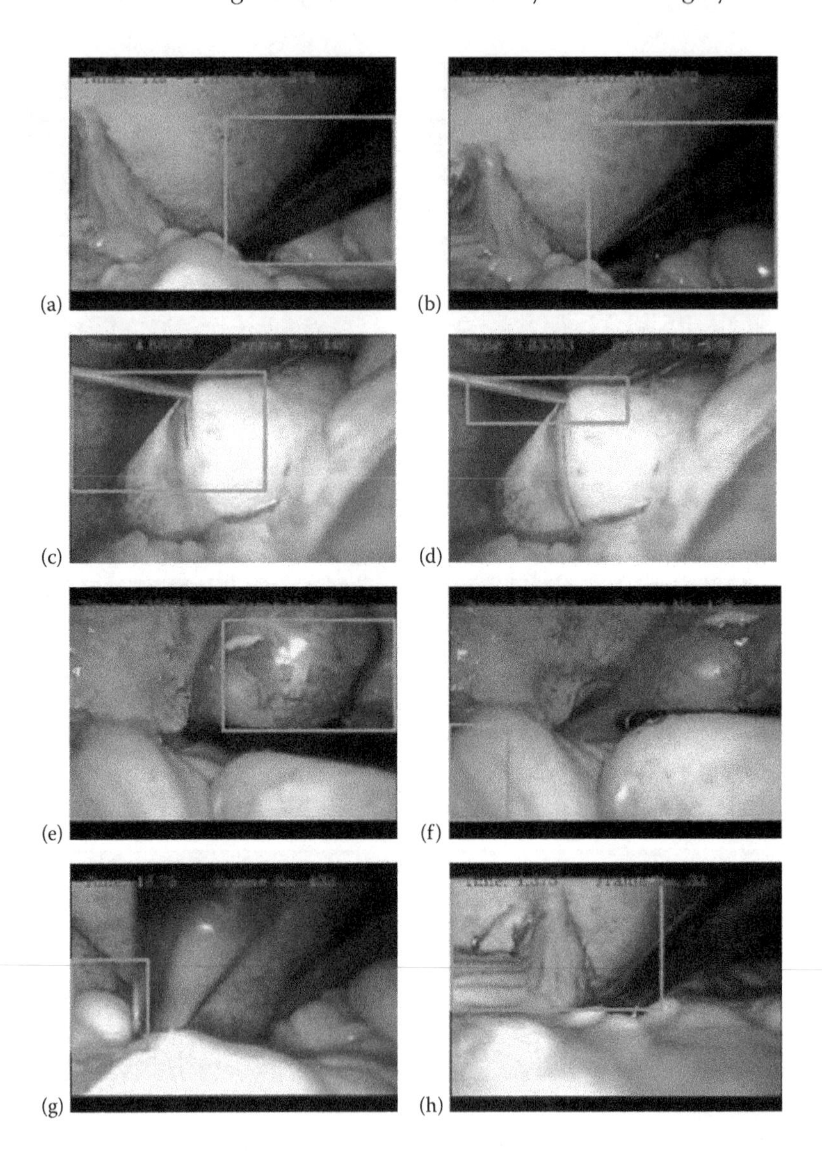

FIGURE 4.31 (a-h) Examples of AGMM surgical tool tracking using endoscopic video of the surgical scene.

laparoscopic reconstruction, accurate motion tracking, and the creation of live images that combine computer-generated graphics with the surgeon's live view of the patient. The use of the AR and 3-D mouse paradigm can significantly facilitate both the learning and performing of minimally invasive interventions in image-guided navigation and surgery. Our initial prototype and *in vitro* experimental evaluations have shown promising results that require further refinement for clinical evaluation.

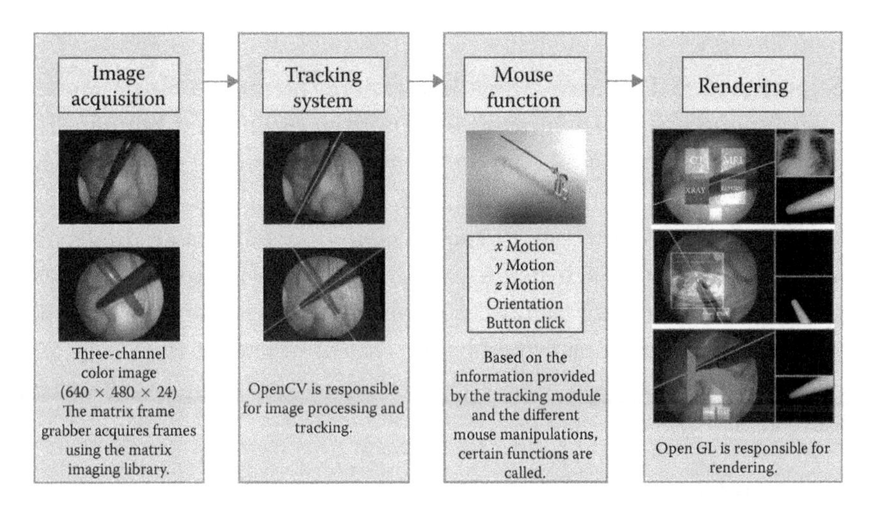

FIGURE 4.32 System architecture for the application of markerless surgical tool tracking for SCI design.

Our current system setup is shown in Figure 4.32. Color images (640 × 480, 24-bit) are acquired from the endoscopic camera. After image acquisition, the tracking subsystem is implemented in three steps: edge extraction, tip localization, and 3-D pose reconstruction. We use a combination of feature-based recognition and the KF process to achieve a robust, reliable instrument tracking. The next step is to perform interactive functions with tool manipulations. The system recognizes the position and orientation of the tool to call a certain function—for example, to click a button or rotate a 3-D virtual cube. The final step of the SCI is to render the virtual environment based on the mouse interactions. The following sections present the last two steps of the overall software architecture, including SCI design and rendering implementation.

Design of an Augmented Surgical Environment

In the previous chapter, two SCIs were presented based on the marker-based framework (i.e., the *ring menu* and the *gesture-based recognition system*). These two interfaces provide an intuitive design; however, neither of them can achieve 3-D manipulation of the overlaid objects using surgical tools. This section presents a comprehensive design that enables surgeons not only to access 2-D images but also to manipulate 3-D medical images of organs. Additionally, the system provides a framework for a two-handed SCI system to manipulate virtual objects—for example, a thread—using two surgical tools.

Menu Design

The proposed SCI contains three levels: *Main menu*, *Submenu*, and an actual function page. Each menu is comprised of different buttons. The main menu contains submenus for *Preoperative images*, *Patient record*, and *3-D effects*. Within each submenu, there are different options. For example, the *Image box* and *Thread manipulation* buttons are under the *3-D effects* submenu. Each submenu provides the option to *Return* to the upper menu or *Exit* the program. A display page is rendered for a specific function call. An example would be the *Patient record* function page and *Image box* function page. An overview of the menu design is shown in Figure 4.33.

Interaction Design

To operate the system, several interactive functions are defined that map the manipulation of the tool to a virtual interaction. All the graphical buttons are designed to be semitransparent. Our interactive system supports the *wait-to-click* paradigm. By tracking the tip

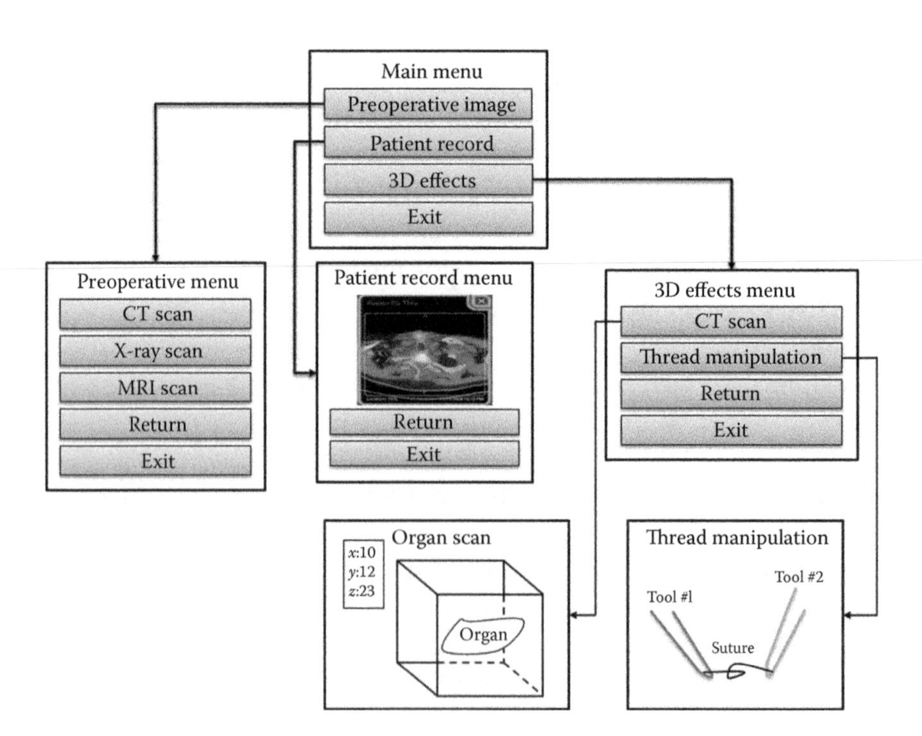

FIGURE 4.33 SCI design and overall structure.

location (i.e., x, y coordinates) of the instrument, certain tasks can be selected. In another words, once the system observes the user pointing the surgical tip (like a cursor) within the area of a button, the button is graphically highlighted. After the button is highlighted for 2 s, the button is considered clicked and the corresponding function is called. Then, the system displays a submenu containing a lower-level set of buttons, such as *CT*, *MRI*, and *X-ray* under the *Preoperative images* menu.

To demonstrate the interactive concept, Figure 4.34a shows the virtual main menu of our proposed SCI, which is comprised of several buttons to direct surgical tasks, including *Preoperative images*, *3-D effects*, and *Patient record*. The left main window shows the tracking result, virtual menus, and objects. The upper-right window shows additional images or patient information and the bottom-right window shows the 3-D-reconstructed tool drawn using OpenGL. For example, in Figure 4.34b, the upper-right window shows the selected x-ray image scan of the patient; in Figure 4.34c, the bottom-right window shows the reconstructed position of the two tools. Additionally, under each submenu or displayed page, the user is able to return to the main menu or exit from the interactive system by clicking the *Return* or *Exit* button.

Figure 4.35 is a display of the *Patient record* function. Critical images and diagnoses are displayed to facilitate surgeons. When necessary, the record will be pulled out from the database and displayed. The designed interface of this function is to translate and move the patient record image according to the tip position. The tip is fixed in the center of the record. Additional information and records can be displayed in the upper-right window.

Figure 4.36 shows the 3-D display of a virtual organ within a cube under the *Image box* function. By selecting one of the faces of the cube (Figure 4.36a), the face is highlighted and it is attached to the surgical tool. The translation of the tip determines the position of the cube in 3-D space (Figure 4.36b).

Figure 4.37 shows the 3-D-augmented display of a virtual surgical suture. By manipulating the suture using two tools, the thread is deformed and translated according to the tips of the tools.

The summary of information/graphical display in the proposed SCI is shown in Table 4.3. As stated previously, the notation (x, y, z) corresponds to the position of the surgical tool tip, and (α, β, γ) to the orientation of the surgical tool.

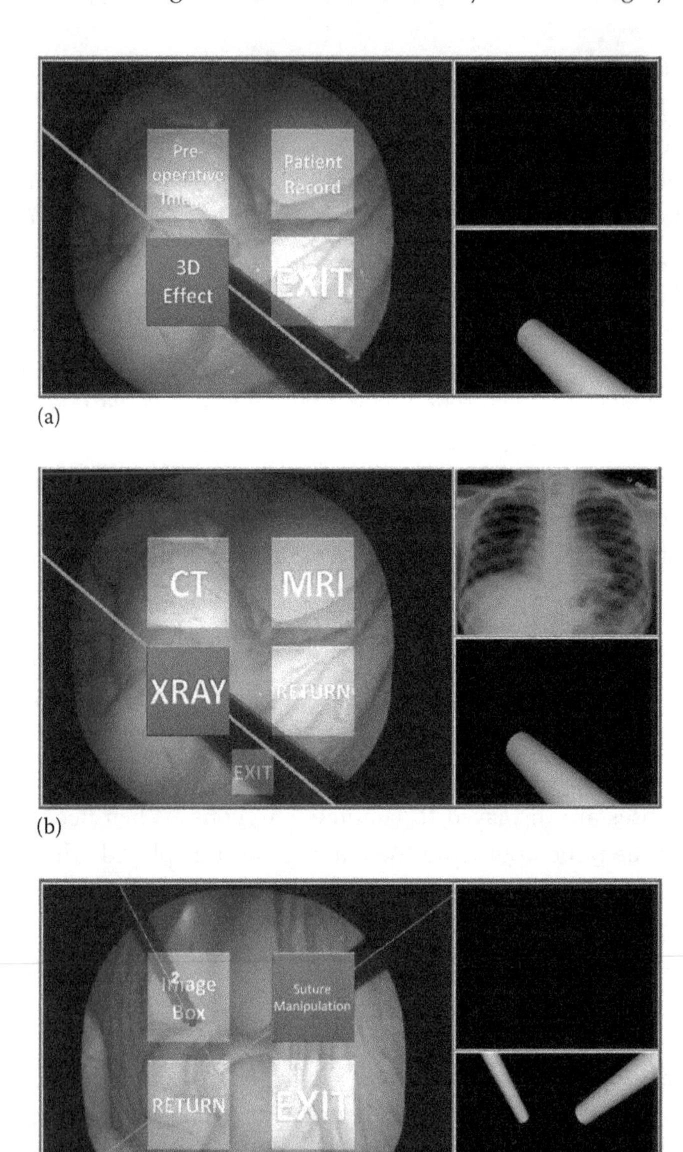

FIGURE 4.34 (a) SCI main menu containing *Preoperative images, Patient record, 3-D effects*, and *Exit*. The *3-D effects* function is selected. (b) Submenus under the *Preoperative images* function, including *CT, MRI, X-ray*, and Return. *X-ray* is selected; the upper-right window shows the x-ray scan once it has been chosen. (c) Submenus under the *3-D effects* function, including *Image box, Suture manipulation, and Return.*

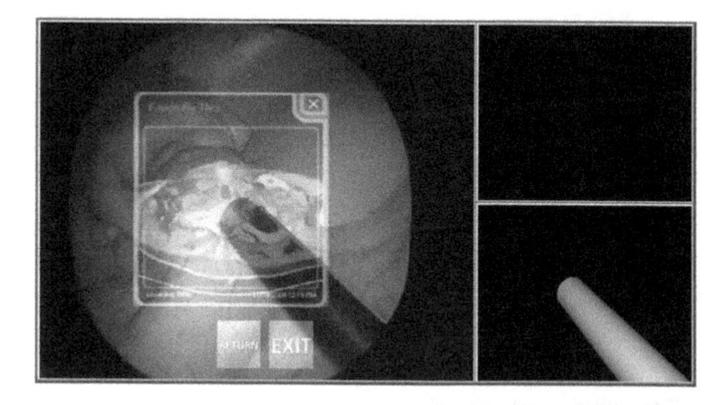

FIGURE 4.35 The *Patient record* function and a demonstration of the notion of image overlay.

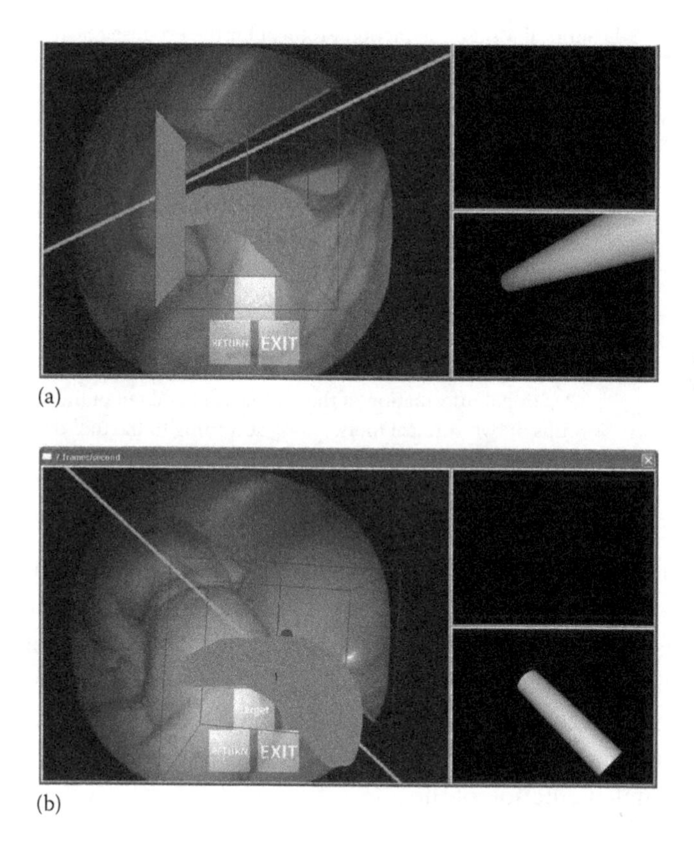

FIGURE 4.36 The *Image box* function. (a) The cube is selected by clicking on one of its faces. (b) The 3-D object can be rotated and translated according to the position of the surgical tool.

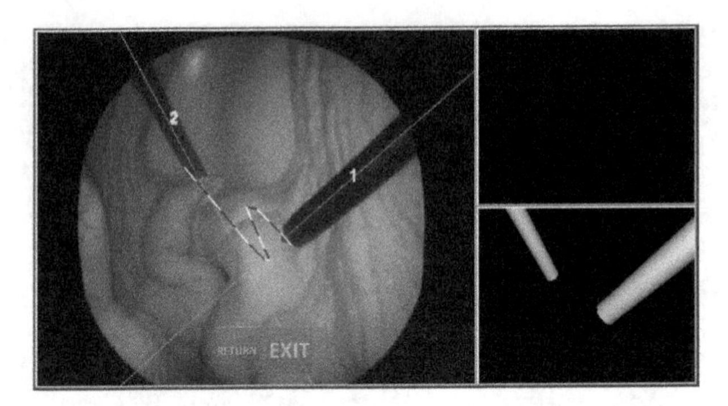

FIGURE 4.37 Augmented *Suture manipulation* function. The suture is manipulated based on the position of the tips. This function is only valid in a two-tool tracking system. The numbers 1 and 2 represent the labels of the tools.

TABLE 4.3 3-D Surgical Mouse Interaction Protocol for the Proposed SCI

Function	Mouse Information	Interaction
Menu Activation	Move the tool tip within the button region.	Wait 2 s and the accordant function is triggered.
Patient medical data	Tip position (x, y, z).	The record sticks to the tip and moves according to the tip location.
Image box function	Tip location is on one of the faces of the cube.	The cube sticks to the tool and the manipulation begins.
	Tip position (x, y, z).	Cube translation in the x, y, z directions.
	Tool orientation (α, β, γ).	Cube rotation along the x, y, z axes.
Suture manipulation	Positional information of the tips of two surgical tools.	The head and tail of the suture moves according to the tool tips.

Implementation of a 3-D Mouse

In order to realize the proposed augmented reality (AR) interactive system for surgical application, the method for graphically displaying the information as a function of the image processing of the surgical tool plays an important role. To align the graphical system with the physical world system, we have to convert camera parameters to OpenGL parameters. This section presents an overview of how this problem is addressed and gives a detailed implementation of the interaction model.

Aligning the Endoscopic and Virtual Images

In the proposed implementation we have utilized open-source libraries such as OpenCV and OpenGL. To allow all the libraries to be compatible with each other, the pixel format needs to be considered in order to render the processed image and virtual graphics. Parameter associations between the graphical display and the virtual endoscopic camera display also need to be considered. Since the 3-D graphics libraries, such as OpenGL, do not use the same parameters for rendering a virtual scene, the intrinsic and extrinsic parameters of a endoscopic camera cannot be directly applied to the virtual object augmentation. The following section presents the relationship between the physical and virtual camera parameters and provides a solution to align the real world to the virtual entities.

The physical camera model has a right-hand coordinate system, as shown in Figure 4.38a. As stated in the previous chapter, this projection relationship can be written as the following equation, assuming the optical center of the camera is the origin of the world frame:

$$u_{\text{real}} = f_x \frac{X}{Z} + u_0 \qquad v_{\text{real}} = f_y \frac{Y}{Z} + v_0 \tag{4.28}$$

For the virtual camera implemented in OpenGL, the coordinate system is defined such that the front of the camera is pointing in the $-Z$ direction.

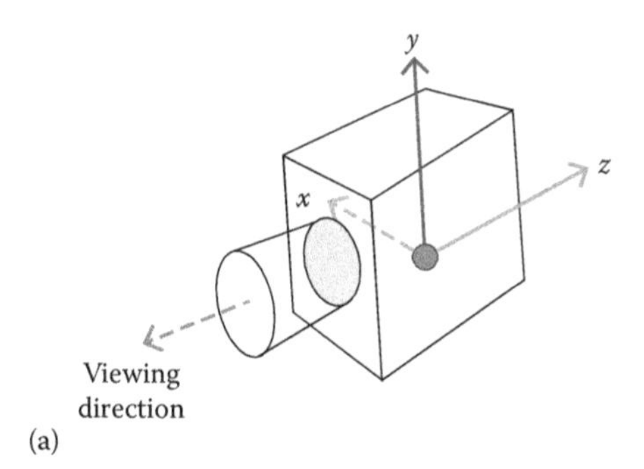

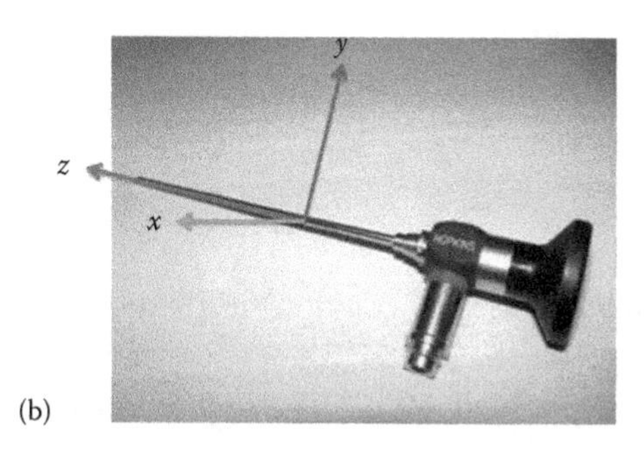

FIGURE 4.38 (a) The camera; (b) the OpenGL reference coordinate frames.

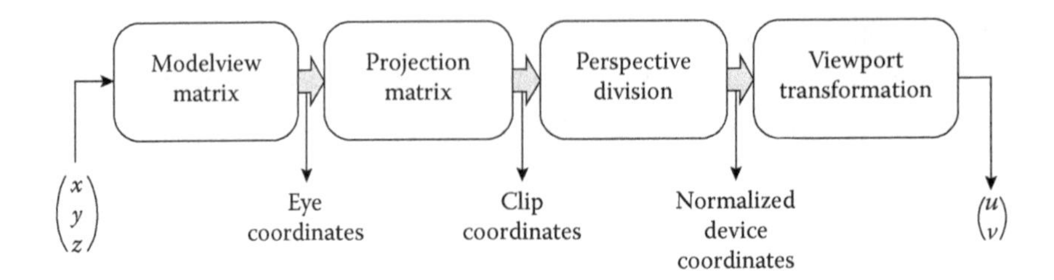

FIGURE 4.39 The OpenGL transformation pipeline.

The $+Y$ direction is the upward vector of the camera. The OpenGL frame is shown in Figure 4.38b. In OpenGL, a 3-D location is transformed to a 2-D image pixel through the following transformation (Guha 2015) (Figure 4.39).

The *Modelview matrix* transforms a 3-D vertex to *eye coordinates*, which is the same as a camera's local coordinates. Thus, the Modelview matrix corresponds to the extrinsic *parameters* of a physical camera. Since the *world frame* is defined at the optical center of the camera, only a definition of the *projection matrix* is needed, which is used to transform the vertex in the eye coordinates system to the *clip coordinates*. The *gluPerspective* function is used here to set up our virtual camera. The syntax of the function call is *gluPerspective (fovy, aspect, Near, Far)*. There are four parameters for the gluPerspective function: *fovy*, *aspect*, *Near*, and *Far*. The transformation matrix can be written as

$$M_p = \begin{bmatrix} \dfrac{\cot\left(\dfrac{f_{ovy}}{2}\right)}{aspect} & 0 & 0 & 0 \\ 0 & \cot\left(\dfrac{f_{ovy}}{2}\right) & 0 & 0 \\ 0 & 0 & \dfrac{zFar + zNear}{zFar - zNear} & \dfrac{2 \cdot zFar \cdot zNear}{zNear - zFar} \\ 0 & 0 & -1 & 0 \end{bmatrix} \quad (4.29)$$

Finally, the *viewport* transformation needs to be determined in order to render the image on the screen. The viewport transformation is set by the function *glViewport (x0, y0, width, height)*. The corresponding transformation matrix transforms the vertex in the clip coordinates system to *window coordinates*:

$$M_v = \begin{bmatrix} \frac{width}{2} & 0 & \frac{width}{2} + x_0 \\ 0 & \frac{height}{2} & \frac{height}{2} + y_0 \\ 0 & 0 & 1 \end{bmatrix} \tag{4.30}$$

The OpenGL setup is completed by multiplying all the matrices together:

$$\begin{bmatrix} u \\ v \\ 1 \end{bmatrix} = M_v \cdot M_p \cdot \begin{bmatrix} X \\ Y \\ Z \end{bmatrix}$$

Finally, we can compute the pixel coordinates of a 3-D point in OpenGL as

$$u_{\text{virtual}} = -\frac{\cot\left(\frac{f_{ovy}}{2}\right) \cdot width \cdot X}{2 \cdot aspect \cdot Z} + \frac{width}{2} + x_0$$

$$v_{\text{virtual}} = -\frac{\cot\left(\frac{f_{ovy}}{2}\right) \cdot height \cdot Y}{2 \cdot aspect \cdot Z} + \frac{height}{2} + y_0 \tag{4.31}$$

Another step needs to be addressed before we can associate and augment the virtual and real-world entities. The OpenGL coordinates are rotated with respect to the image coordinate. For example, the coordinates (0, 0, 1) in the physical camera correspond to (0, 0, −1) in the virtual camera; due to the constraints of the right-hand coordinate system, our image coordinate system is different. Given the virtual and actual pixel coordinates and the frame relationship, we can equate the two correspondences together as

$$f_x \frac{X}{Z} + u_0 = \frac{\cot\left(\frac{f_{ovy}}{2}\right) \cdot width \cdot X}{2 \cdot aspect \cdot Z} + \frac{width}{2} + x_0$$

$$f_y \frac{Y}{Z} + v_0 = \frac{\cot\left(\frac{f_{ovy}}{2}\right) \cdot height \cdot Y}{2 \cdot aspect \cdot Z} + \frac{height}{2} - y_0 \tag{4.32}$$

Three-Dimensional Manipulation of Augmented Virtual Images

The *Image box* function is developed in order to simulate a system that superimposes 3-D preoperative images on the top of a physical object. This can be used for various image-guided surgical diagnostics and procedures. Examples would be to access and display information on the graphical entities, zoom in on the virtual object, and access live scans in order to visualize abnormal tissue or a tumor. The proposed design would allow the surgeon to translate, scale, and rotate the virtual organ containing the medical information/images. To simplify the design, we assume that the organ is enclosed by a cube. Hence, through manipulation of the cube, the organ is moved accordingly. Another example of this application is to help surgeons manually register the preoperative scan on a real organ. Since the preoperative scans and live endoscopic images of the organ are not necessarily taken from the same viewing perspective, the surgeon might use the system to superimpose the scan on top of the live images to enhance the visualization during MIS.

As shown in Figure 4.36, the program allows the user to click one face of the virtual cube with the surgical tool to start the manipulation. The cube is originally drawn at a depth of 80 mm away from the camera. The length is 40 mm with zero rotation around its axis. In order to have a natural way of displaying the virtual objects, the interface preserves the perspective view of the cube. In another words, the cube becomes smaller as it moves farther away and larger as it moves nearer to the camera.

When the surgical tool moves close to the vicinity of one of its faces, the face is highlighted. If the user holds the tool for another 2 s, the face is clicked and sticks to the tool tip. This means that the grabbed box will shift with the tool tip and the organ inside the cube will move accordingly.

In order to control the cube movement, the cube manipulation is divided into translation and rotation parts along the x, y, and z axes in the camera frame. Both translation and rotation are based on the start pose of the tool as $T_o(x_o, y_o, z_o)$ and $R_o(\alpha_o, \beta_o, \gamma_o)$. As the manipulation begins, the new pose of the tool in the nth frame becomes $T_n(x_n, y_n, z_n)$ and $R_n(\alpha_n, \beta_n, \gamma_n)$. The cube translation and rotation along each axis are as follows:

$$
\begin{aligned}
T_n^{cube} &= T_n - T_o = \left(x_n - x_o, y_n - y_o, z_n - z_o\right) \\
R_n^{cube} &= R_n - R_o = \left(\alpha_n - \alpha_o, \beta_n - \beta_o, \gamma_n - \gamma_o\right)
\end{aligned}
\tag{4.33}
$$

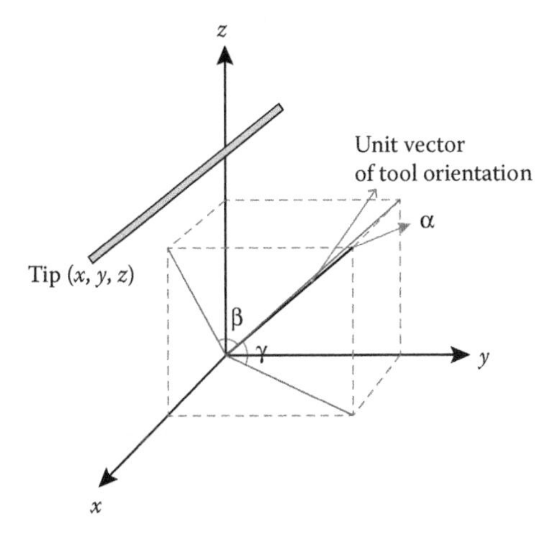

FIGURE 4.40 Notation of the tool tip $T(x, y, z)$ and rotation angle $R(\alpha, \beta, \gamma)$.

where T is the position of the tool tip and R is the including angle of the tool orientation vector with respect to the YZ, XZ, and XY surfaces, respectively (as shown in Figure 4.40).

The orientation angles are calculated from the following equation:

$$\alpha = \arctan\left(\frac{x}{\sqrt{y^2+z^2}}\right) \beta = \arctan\left(\frac{y}{\sqrt{x^2+z^2}}\right) \gamma = \arctan\left(\frac{z}{\sqrt{x^2+y^2}}\right) \tag{4.34}$$

By manipulating the tool, the virtual organ can be zoomed in and out by translating the tool on the Z axis. It can also be rotated by moving the tool vector in different directions. For example, in order to demonstrate the notion of the organ registration, a *target* positioning can be initiated by pressing the button located at the handle of the surgical tool (Figure 4.41) (Sun and Payandeh 2011a,b).

By manipulating the cube, the user can place the organ to align with the target organ, as shown in Figure 4.42. As will be shown in Chapter 6, it is possible to define a target image that is anchored to the actual surgical site using various feature points. When the graphical markers representing the axes of the overlaid organ are within distance of the anchored target markers, the two objects can be overlaid (Figure 4.42d).

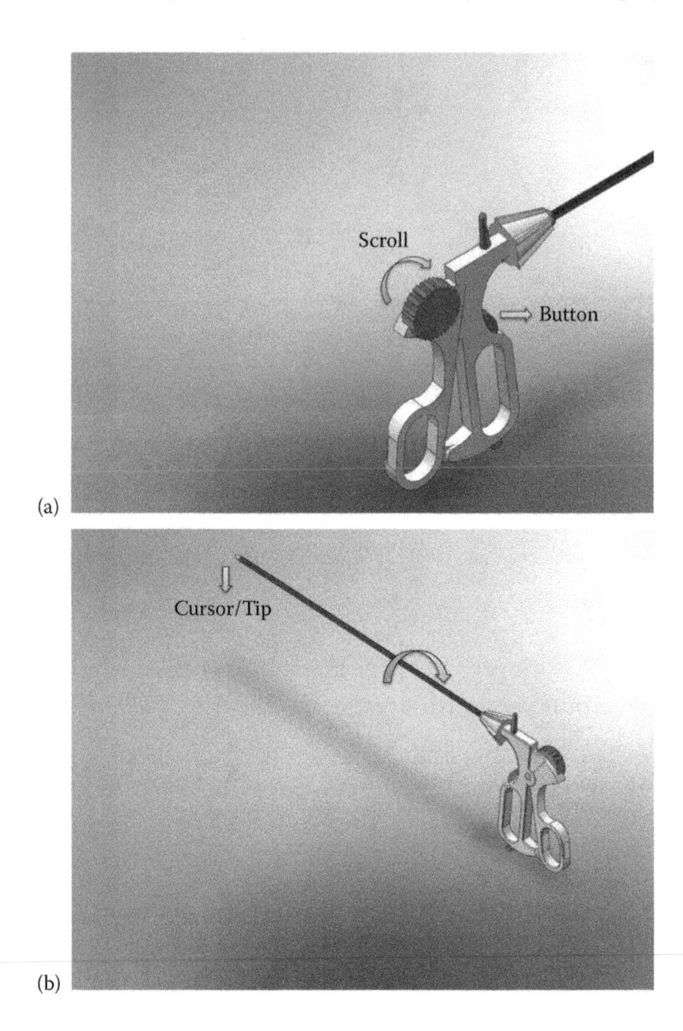

FIGURE 4.41 Design of the surgical tool: (a) a standard scroll wheel and button can be added to the handle; (b) association of the surgical tool motion to that of the motion of the tool tip.

Two-Handed Manipulation of a Virtual Suture

The *Suture manipulation* function simulates a suture and a suturing task, where two tools work as two needles to manipulate the thread. This is one of the most complex examples of developing an AR, where the graphical objects are described by difference equations (LeDuc et al. 2003; Payandeh and Shi 2010). The single-dimension mass-spring model is used to model the sutures and the strings. The behavior of the string is dominated by the internal forces acting on each mass point or element. The internal forces include the friction force, linear spring, linear damper, tensional spring,

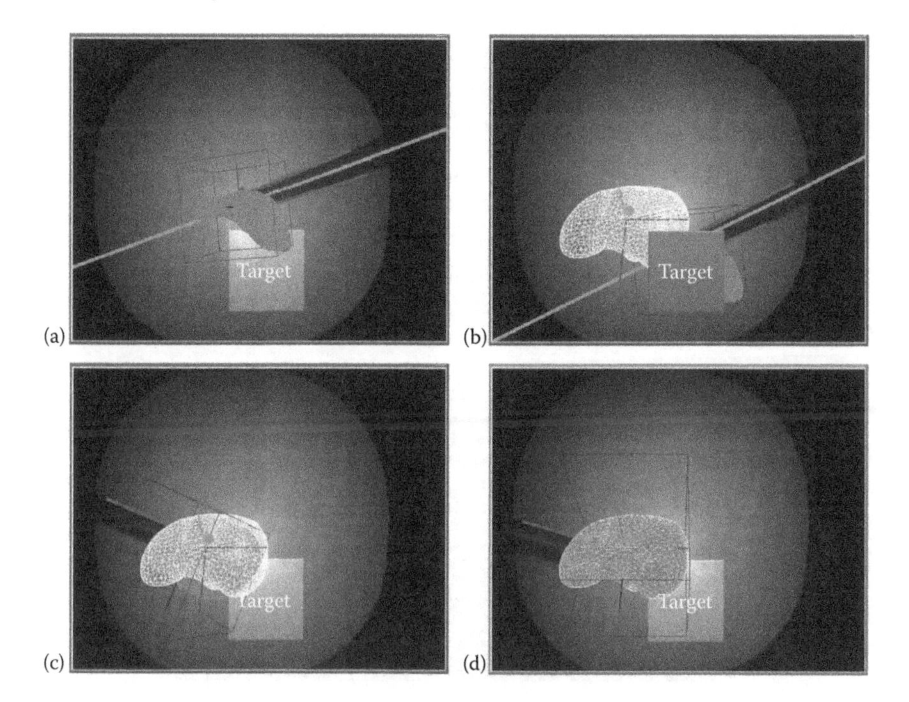

FIGURE 4.42 (a-d) Screenshots of the tool manipulation procedure to register a virtual organ to the target.

tensional damper, and swivel damper. Various behaviors of the suture can be modeled, such as bending and twisting or knotting and unknotting. During graphical rendering, the cylinders as suture segments are connected to each other between two successive points. The shape of the suture is calculated using the explicit Euler method. The screenshots in Figure 4.43 show samples of suture manipulation using two surgical tools, involving stretching, pulling, and crossing.

SUMMARY

This chapter has presented a new tracking framework based on the KF (Gaussian-based) approach and its various extensions. Unlike the methodology of the previous chapter, the visual tracking does not rely on any engineered marker placed on the surgical tool or any stored patterns that can be recognized as a gesture. The method of this chapter utilizes more common feature-based detection algorithms. The combination of these top-down and bottom-up approaches can provide a robust system with multiple surgical tool tracking capabilities. To track the surgical tool, three Gaussian-type methods, KF, EKF, and AGMM, have been presented in this

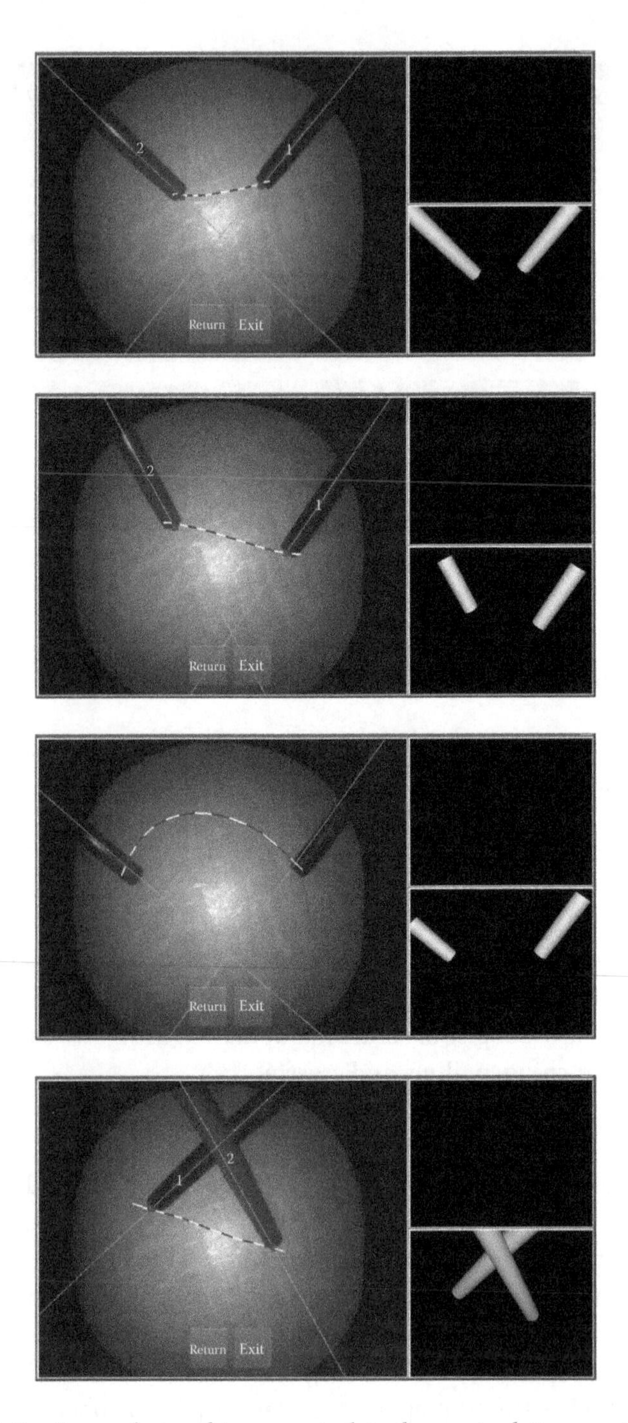

FIGURE 4.43 Screenshots of two surgical tools manipulating a virtual augmented suture.

chapter. The experiments were conducted in both an *in vitro* environment and an *in vivo* environment. In the *in vitro* experiment, all three methods were able deal with single surgical instrument tracking. Compared with the KF and the EKF methods, the AGMM is more robust with respect to noise. The chapter has also shown how the spatial description of the surgical tool can be used in augmentation with the 3-D graphical objects. A method for calibrating both the visual track information and the graphical model has been presented. Various notions of image-guided manipulation and guidance through augmented reality have also been explored in order to form the basis for future design and development.

CHAPTER 5

Markerless Tracking: Non-Gaussian Approach

THE GAUSSIAN-TYPE TRACKING METHODS presented in the previous chapter—Kalman filter (KF), extended Kalman filter (EKF), and adaptive Gaussian mixture model (AGMM)—are based on the assumption that the nature of exogenous inputs to the tracking system (i.e., input disturbances and reference tracking) exhibit normal or Gaussian properties. In addition, it is assumed that the dynamic model of the system, which models the propagation of the state between samples, follows a linear model.

It can also be stated that in minimally invasive surgery (MIS), the motion of the surgical tools that are being held by the surgeon also exhibit non-Gaussian and nonlinear properties. This is due to the nature of the surgical procedure and the movement intentions of the surgeon at each time interval. This chapter explores a tracking scheme that can capture both the nonlinear and non-Gaussian properties of the motions associated with the movements of surgical tools. The particle filter (PF), which belongs to the non-Gaussian-type tracking framework, has been used in various tracking problems associated with people and vehicles (Yang et al. 2010; Khong et al. 2011; Lee and Payandeh 2015).

In this chapter, we present the PF and its modified implementation as visual tracking algorithms. In the modified implementation, a weight-based resampling strategy can be adapted for tracking the motion of the surgical tools that are being held by the surgeon. Moreover, a hybrid approach that combines both the PF framework and the AGMM is implemented for tracking, which provides two-dimensional (2-D) information regarding the features of the surgical tool. These methods are experimentally evaluated in both an *in vitro* scene and an *in vivo* video stream, and are also compared with the Gaussian-type methods that were presented in the previous chapter.

REVIEW OF PARTICLE FILTER

Particle filter, also called the *sequential Monte Carlo* method, is a tracking approach to estimate the posterior density distribution of the state of the tracked object based on a set of Bayesian recursive equations. In addition to the previous Gaussian and linear assumptions, the PF is able to solve the tracking problem in a nonlinear dynamical environment with a non-Gaussian density model (Ristic et al. 2004).

The basic framework of the PF is to generate a group of weighted samples that can be used to approximate the posterior probability density function (PDF) of the state of the tracked dynamical system. These samples are called *particles* and they are weighted according to the weighting function based on metrics associated with the measurements. For example, for visual tracking problems, the weight function is created on the basis of measurements from the image data captured through the endoscopic imaging system. If some samples are more reliable than others, they are given higher weights according to the function, so that the new propagated particles have a tendency to be more concentrated around those reliable particles. In general, if the number of particles is large enough, we can recover the unknown posterior PDF of the state of the tracked dynamical system using its approximation after several iterations (Appendix III).

As was mentioned, since the PF method does not assume any linearity of the system or Gaussian distribution of noise, it is widely used in object-tracking problems such as people tracking (Breitenstein et al. 2009) and vehicle tracking (Tehrani Niknejad et al. 2012). PF has also been implemented in medical and surgical applications—for example, in tracking a capsule endoscope's location (Anzai and Wang 2013) and in identifying cancerous or bleeding regions (Sousa et al. 2009; Li and Meng 2009). A color-based PF method was also applied for people tracking in a multicamera surveillance system (Lu 2008). A similar PF method was used to track a colored marker in an emulated surgical scene (Sun and Payandeh 2011a,b). To explore the method for markerless tracking in MIS applications, a modified PF framework is proposed in order to determine the possible region of a moving surgical instrument. Based on this region, further feature detection steps are carried out in order to locate the edges and tip of the surgical tool.

Similar to the KF and the EKF, the PF framework is also a recursive Bayesian estimator based on Monte Carlo simulation. For the visual-tracking problem, the state of the process, which is represented by a state vector, should contain the relevant information about the target that we would like to track. For example, in the previous chapter, the state vector of the KF method is defined from the midline description of the surgical tool, and the state vector description for the EKF method is defined based on the description of the two edges of the surgical tool. In the case of visual tracking using a PF, a region within the scene that contains the surgical tool is selected for tracking purposes. In comparison with the feature-based approach used in the previous chapter, the region-based approach offers reduced sensitivity of the tracking to the surrounding images. In the implementation, the target object is selected to be the rectangular region (e.g., *Rec*) that indicates the possible area for the surgical tool.

Let us define a set of samples, $S = \left\{\left(s_t^{(i)}, \pi_t^{(i)}\right) | i = 1,\ldots,N\right\}$, with associated weights $\pi_t^{(i)}$. Let the estimate of current state M_t—namely, $E(M_t)$—be computed based on these samples and weights. As the number of samples grows, the PF can recover the true posterior PDF. Let the system dynamic model be defined as

$$M_t = F_t\left(M_{t-1}, w_{t-1}\right) \tag{5.1}$$

where F_t is a possibly nonlinear function of the previous state and process noise. The set of samples is propagated according to the system dynamic model as

$$s_t^{(i)} = F_t\left(s_{t-1}^{(i)}, w_{t-1}\right) \tag{5.2}$$

Each sample in the set is weighted by the normalized probability

$$\pi_t^{(i)} = p\left(z_t | M_t = s_t^{(i)}\right), \quad \left(\sum_{i=1}^{N} \pi_t^{(i)} = 1\right) \tag{5.3}$$

where z_t is the observation at time t. Therefore, the estimated state vector at time t can be defined as

$$E(M_t) = \sum_{i=1}^{N} \pi_t^{(i)} s_t^{(i)} \tag{5.4}$$

As stated, the approach is also referred to as *recursive Bayesian filtering by Monte Carlo simulations*. The recursion operates in two phases: prediction and update. The evolution of the sample set is propagated in each sample according to the system model (prediction). Each element of the set is then weighted in terms of the observations (update phase). Here we explore a number of implementations of the PF for tracking surgical tools.

Example Implementations of Particle Filter

An ellipse is used to define a region on the image, similar to the shape defined in Figure 5.1.

The state vector representation of the shape of this region can be defined as

$$x_t^{(i)} = \left[x, y, \dot{x}, \dot{y}, H_x, H_y, \theta\right]_t^T \tag{5.5}$$

where:

- (x, y) specifies the location of the ellipse
- $(\dot{x}, \dot{y})$ is the velocity
- H_x and H_y are the radius of the ellipse used to represent the marker in both directions
- θ is the rotation of the marker, or the surgical tool, in the image plane

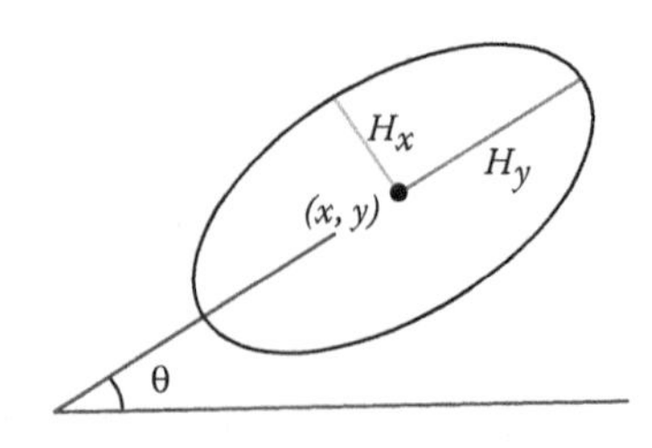

FIGURE 5.1 Ellipse presentation of a region on the image of the surgical tool tip.

From Equation 5.1, the prediction or propagation is assumed to have the following form:

$$x_t^{(i)} = Ax_{t-1}^{(i)} + Rw_{t-1} \tag{5.6}$$

The update stage is to reweight the samples by observation. To determine the color distribution inside the elliptical region, the color histogram from each of the HSV channels of the camera is computed (Nummiaro et al. 2003). At each iteration cycle, the samples need to be reweighted according to the likelihood by comparing the color distribution template within m bins. Here, the likelihood function between two distributions $p^{(u)}$ and $q^{(u)}$ ($u = 1, 2, \ldots, m$) is determined by calculating the Bhattacharyya coefficient:

$$\rho[p,q] = \sum_{u=1}^{m} \sqrt{p^{(u)} q^{(u)}} \tag{5.7}$$

A small Bhattacharyya distance corresponds to large weights. The magnitude of weight can be updated by a Gaussian model with variance σ as

$$\pi^{(i)} = \frac{1}{\sqrt{2\pi\sigma}} e^{(\rho[p,q]-1)/2\sigma^2} \tag{5.8}$$

Figure 5.2 shows an overall diagram of the basic implementation of the color-based particle filter.

Figure 5.3 shows a comparison study between the moving history image (MHI) and the PF at various frames of the visual-tracking procedure. In this experiment, 100 particles were selected (Sun and Payandeh 2011a).

In another implementation of color-based particle filtering for tracking surgical tools, the initial geometrical region obtained through MHI is used for defining the tracking state variable at time t:

$$x_t^{(i)} = [x_C, y_C, x'_C, y'_C, w_R, h_R, w'_R, h'_R]_t^T \tag{5.9}$$

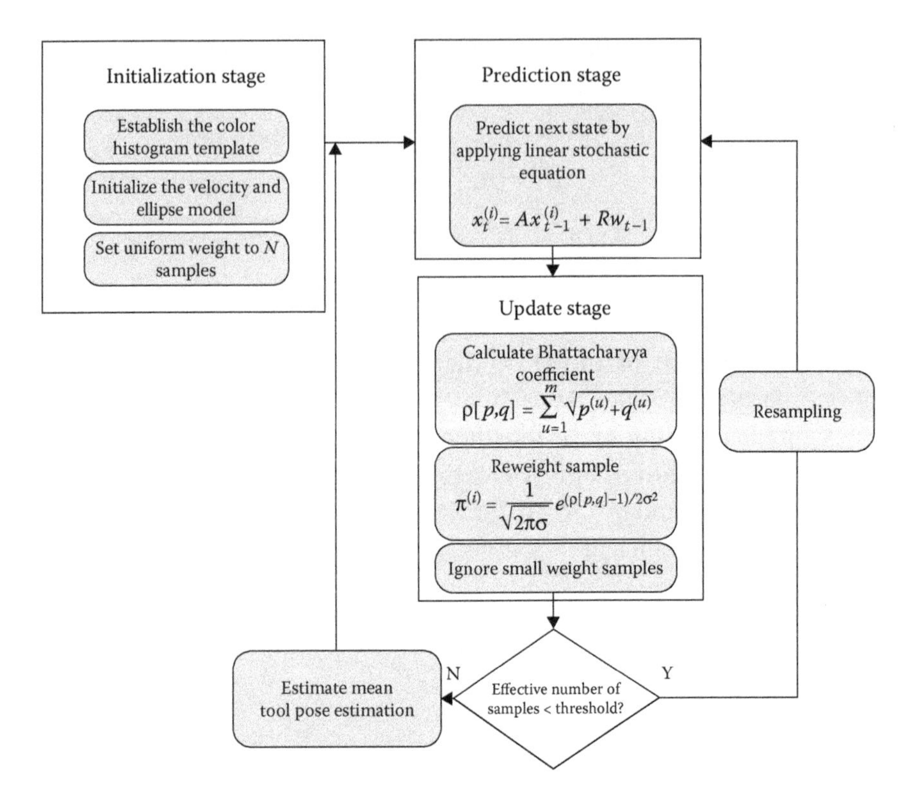

FIGURE 5.2 Implementation of the color-based PF.

where:

(x_C, y_C)	are the center coordinates of the rectangular region
w_R and h_R	are the width and height of the rectangle
x'_C and y'_C	are the time rate of change of the coordinates of the center point along the x and y directions
w'_R and h'_R	are the instantaneous changes of width and height of the rectangular region

Similar to the previous implementation of the PF, in order to estimate the target area in the image, some measured variables are needed. These variables are from the image data obtained through the endoscope imaging system. They are used as measurements for our tracking setup, which will be tracking the surgical tool during the operation. Through experimental observations, it was found that the color distribution in the surgical scene and the tracking region where the surgical tool could

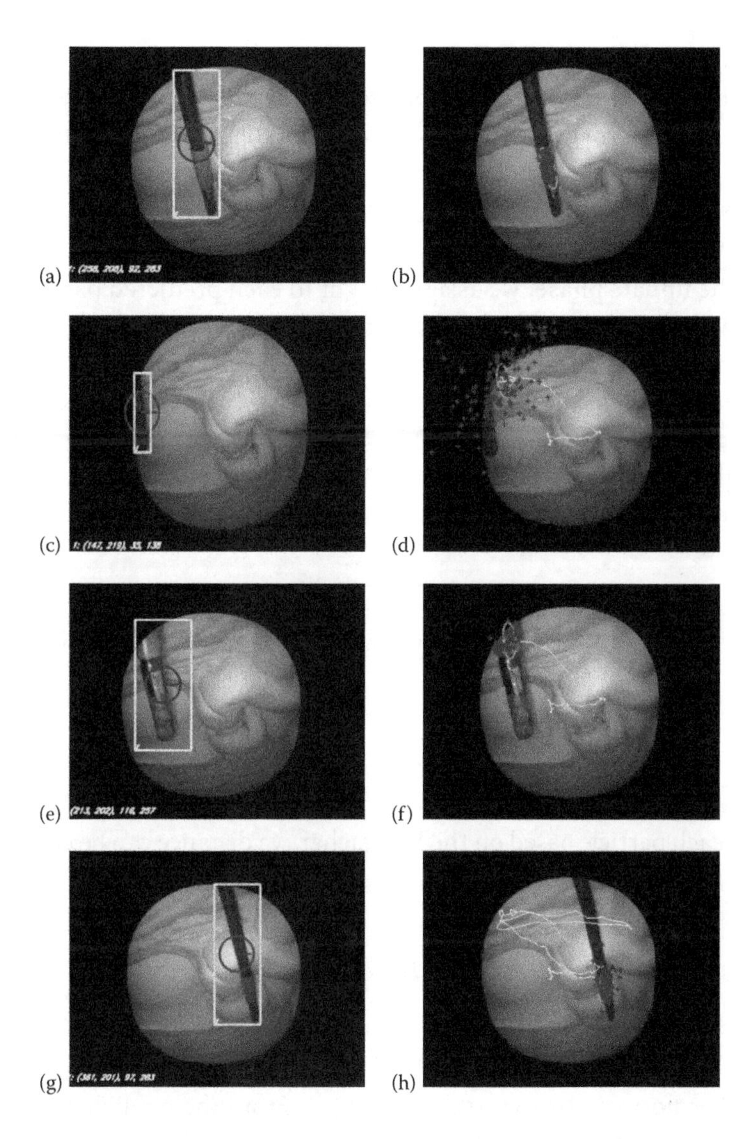

FIGURE 5.3 (a-h) Comparison between the PF and MHI results. The first column of images shows single tool tracking by using MHI-based tracking. The rectangle represents the bonding box of the whole object and the circular dial represents the motion flow. The second column of images shows the tracking results by applying the PF. The ellipse represents the expected object location. Dots are the distributed particles. The curves record the trajectory of the object. By tracking the red marker, we can trace the desired marker efficiently.

be located tend to have more dark or bright components in comparison with other regions. In comparison with other color spaces such as RGB and gray scale, the hue, saturation, and value (HSV) space has better tracking performance under different illumination conditions because the illumination and color information are stored in two bins (channels).

In the update phase, we assign weight to each predicted particle $x_t^{(i)}$ by comparing the 2-D histogram of the current sample area with the reference histogram. The reference histogram comes from the target region defined in the initialization step (or consecutive stages). An expanded version of Equation 5.7 for computing the distance between two histograms of particle i and the reference histogram can be written as

$$d_B = \sqrt{1 - \sum_{j=1}^{M} \sqrt{hist^i[j] \cdot hist_{ref}[j]}} \quad \text{with} \quad M = m_{Hbin} \times m_{Sbin} \tag{5.10}$$

where m_{Hbin} and m_{Sbin} are the numbers of storage bins for hue and saturation, respectively. In this implementation of particle filtering, the weight $w[i]$ of each particle based on the Bhattacharyya distance can be computed as

$$w[i] = e^{-\lambda d_B^2} \tag{5.11}$$

where λ is an empirically determined coefficient. This weighting function is further normalized to satisfy $\sum_{i=1}^{N} w[i]=1$. From the predicted particles and their weights, we can estimate the possible region for the moving surgical instrument using their expected value $E(x_t) = \sum_{i=1}^{N} w_t^{(i)} s_t^{(i)}$. This value is used to determine the tracking result at current time t.

One of the drawbacks of implementing a PF is its degeneracy problem. In practice and after a few iterations, all but one of the normalized weights tend toward zero. To avoid this phenomenon, a resampling step is required to eliminate particles with low weight values. For example, an effective sample size can be defined to be used as a criterion for identifying if the resampling step is necessary. The effective sample size N_{eff} is defined as

$$N_{eff} = \frac{1}{\sum_{i=1}^{N} w^{(i)^2}} \tag{5.12}$$

If N_{eff} is lower than a given threshold N_{th}, the particles can be resampled following a predefined methodology, and the new generated particles are used as the input posterior PDF for the next time, $t+1$.

MODIFICATION TO THE RESAMPLING STRATEGY

In the PF, the resampling step plays a significant part in finding the best approximation to the posterior PDF. In the previous implementation of the PF framework (Lu 2008), the new particles are randomly resampled from the predicted particle sets. This method does not take into account the weight information, which makes the propagation of the particles trivial in having a sparse distribution. Here it is proposed that particles with higher weights should be considered more reliable in comparison with others. Based on this observation, an alternative adaptive resampling strategy is presented.

In the proposed adaptive resampling strategy, first the predicted particles are sorted in descending order, $\{s^{(1)}, s^{(2)}, \ldots, s^{(N)}\}$, according to their weight values, so the particles with higher weights have the priority of being chosen. To generate the new particle set, we take the first element from the particle queue $\{s^{(1)}, s^{(2)}, \ldots, s^{(N)}\}$ and make n_{update} copies of it in the new particle set. The number n_{update} is calculated from the following relationship:

$$n_{\text{update}}[j] = \min\left(h \in Z \mid h \geq n_{\text{update}}[j]\right)$$

$$\sum_{j=1}^{m} n_{\text{update}}[j] = N \tag{5.13}$$

where m is the number of elements we selected from the particle queue. For example, let five particles $\{x^{(1)}, x^{(2)}, x^{(3)}, x^{(4)}, x^{(5)}\}$ be given with weights $\{0.1, 0.5, 0.1, 0.1, 0.2\}$. Firstly, we put the particle queue $\{q^{(1)}, q^{(2)}, q^{(3)}, q^{(4)}, q^{(5)}\}$ in descending order and scan the queue from the beginning. Since the weight for the first element $q^{(1)}$ is 0.5, we make three copies of $q^{(1)}$ in the new particle set $\{x^{*(1)}, x^{*(2)}, x^{*(3)}, x^{*(4)}, x^{*(5)}\}$. Then we move to the second

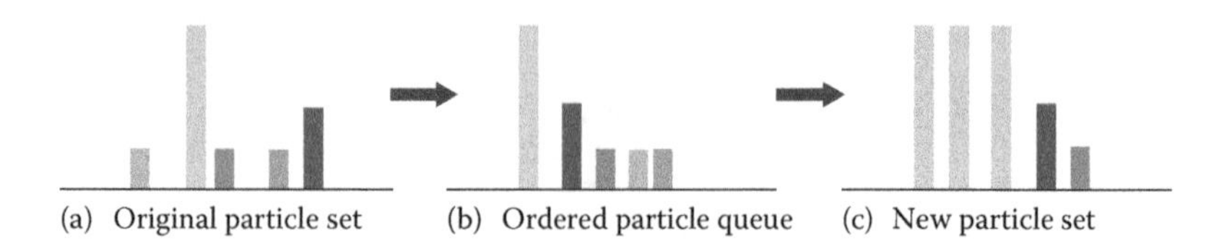

FIGURE 5.4 Illustration of the weight-based resampling strategy. (a) The original particle set has five particles indicated in different colors. The height represents its weight. In (b), the particles are organized in a descending order. After resampling, the new particle set (c) contains the copies from those particles with high weights (green, blue, and gray ones). The particles with low weights (red and orange) are removed from the particle set.

element $q^{(2)}$ and make a copy of it. We do the same step to the remaining elements in the particle queue until we have made enough copies for the new particle sets. As a result, we have the following updated particles:

$$\left\{x^{*(1)}, x^{*(2)}, x^{*(3)}, x^{*(4)}, x^{*(5)}\right\} = \left\{q^{(1)}, q^{(2)}, q^{(3)}, q^{(4)}, q^{(5)}\right\} \tag{5.14}$$

By applying the weight-based strategy, the resampled particle set has a more concentrated distribution around highly weighted regions while neglecting those with low weights. Figure 5.4 illustrates an example of weight-based resampling (Zhou and Payandeh 2015b).

HYBRID APPROACH: INTEGRATING THE PF AND AGMM

In the previous chapter, a Gaussian method was introduced for background subtraction of the surgical tool based on the AGMM approach, which is able to detect a moving foreground object on a stable background. However, in some cases, the approach may not produce acceptable tracking results if the background or the viewing direction of the endoscope is changing. The PF approach has the advantage of solving a nonlinear dynamic system and a non-Gaussian density model, but it requires a definition of the initial state vector (which sometimes requires external activation, such as an activation key attached at the handle of the surgical tool). Similarly, if the tracking is lost, it is hard for the PF to recover the tracking without some other external input. A hybrid method is proposed that integrates the PF and the AGMM. Through the initialization of the tracked region for the PF implementation, 2-D feature detection is applied

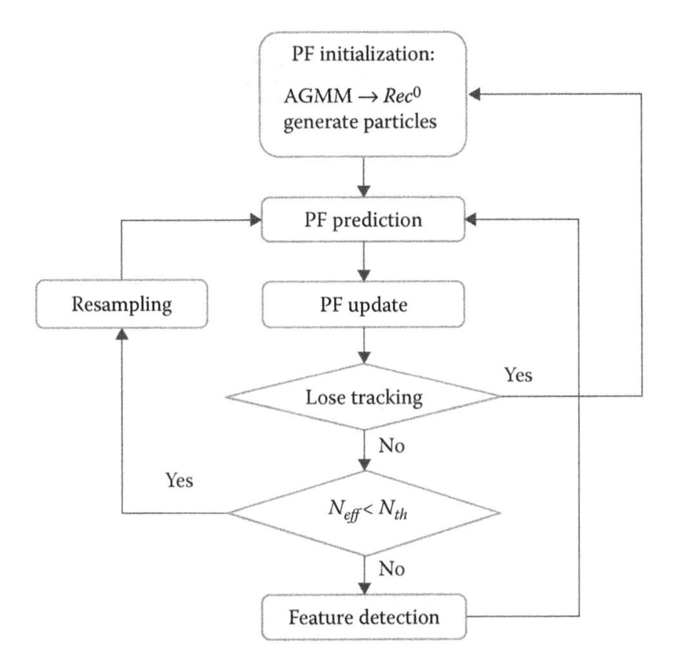

FIGURE 5.5 Flow chart of the hybrid non-Gaussian approach that combines a PF and an AGMM.

within the defined region in order to identify the two edges of the surgical tool and its associated tip.

Figure 5.5 shows a flowchart of the proposed hybrid approach. As stated, the proposed hybrid method replaces this manual initialization with an automatic procedure. For a given video stream, it is first split it into short clips, each of which last only 1–2 s. We assume that the backgrounds in these video clips are relatively stable so that the AGMM is able to detect the moving object. Before we start the PF tracking, the AGMM is first applied to determine the initial position of the moving surgical tool, which returns a rectangular region containing the tool. We use this rectangular region to compute the reference histogram and to generate particles in the initialization of the PF. After the initialization, the PF is then responsible for tracking the surgical tool. If the tracking is lost, the AGMM is applied again to relocate the rectangular region that encloses the initial position of surgical tool, and the PF is reinitialized.

After we obtain the region of interest from the PF, we use the feature detection method introduced in the previous chapter to find the tip position of the surgical tool. The Canny edge detector and the Hough

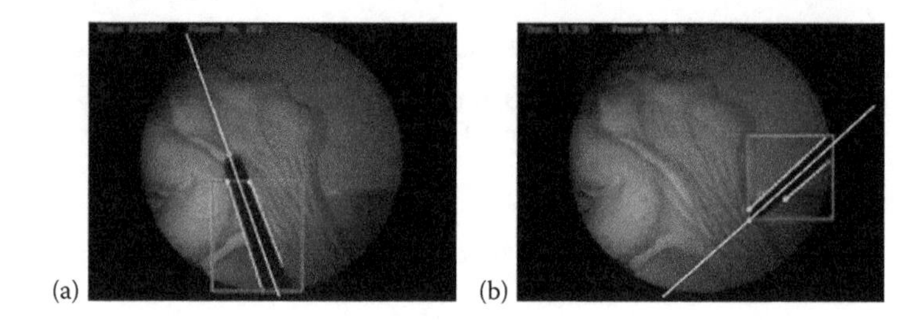

FIGURE 5.6 Demonstration of tracking using the hybrid method: (a) and (b) are the tracking results in different positions. The rectangle indicates the region of interest returned from the PF framework, and two edges of the tool are labeled by short line segments. The small circle refers to the tool's tip and the center line is the midline of the tool.

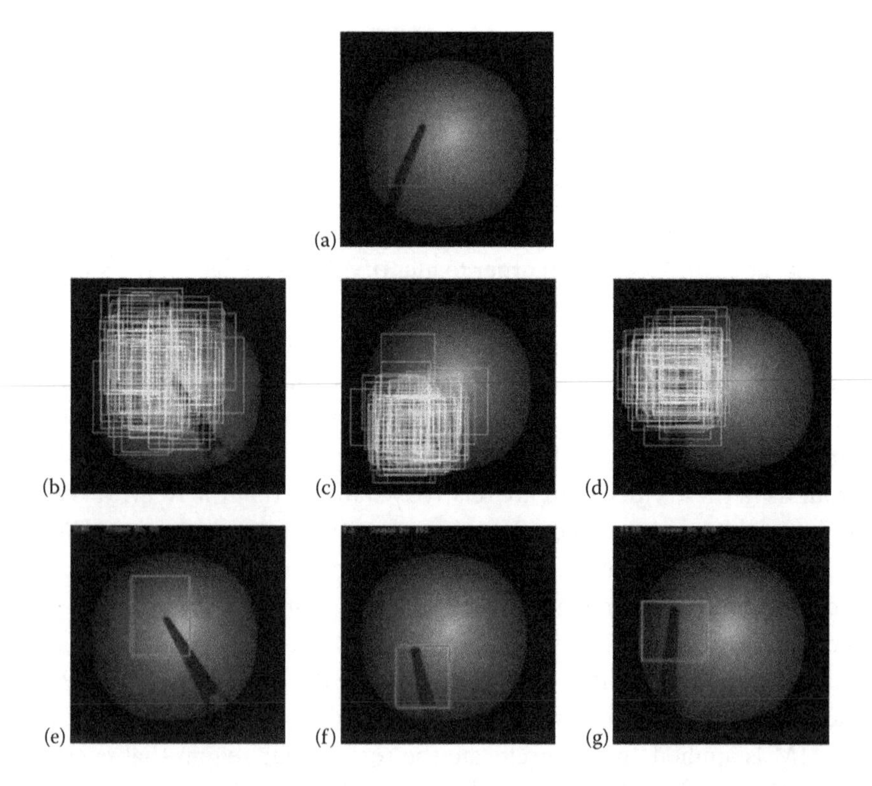

FIGURE 5.7 Tracking results of the modified PF approach in an ideal *in vitro* scene. The initial region is defined in (a); (b), (c), and (d) are the generated particles at different times; (e), (f), and (g) are the tracking results corresponding to (b), (c), and (d).

transform are applied within the region that is being tracked. The detected line segments are classified into two groups according to their relative distances. The line segments in the same group are merged to form the edge of the surgical tool. From the extracted two edges, we can calculate the midline of the tool and represent it in the slope intercept form $y = mx + b$. We search along the midline to find the point with the largest intensity change, which is considered the tool's tip. Figure 5.6 demonstrates the tracking result by using the hybrid tracking method.

EXPERIMENTAL STUDIES

Similar to the Gaussian-type tracking experiments, the modified PF method and the hybrid method were both evaluated in *in vitro* and *in vivo* environments. The number of particles for the PF and for the hybrid method was selected to be 100. During the tracking, the user can adjust the parameters of the Canny detector and the Hough transform in order to identify the best feature detection result.

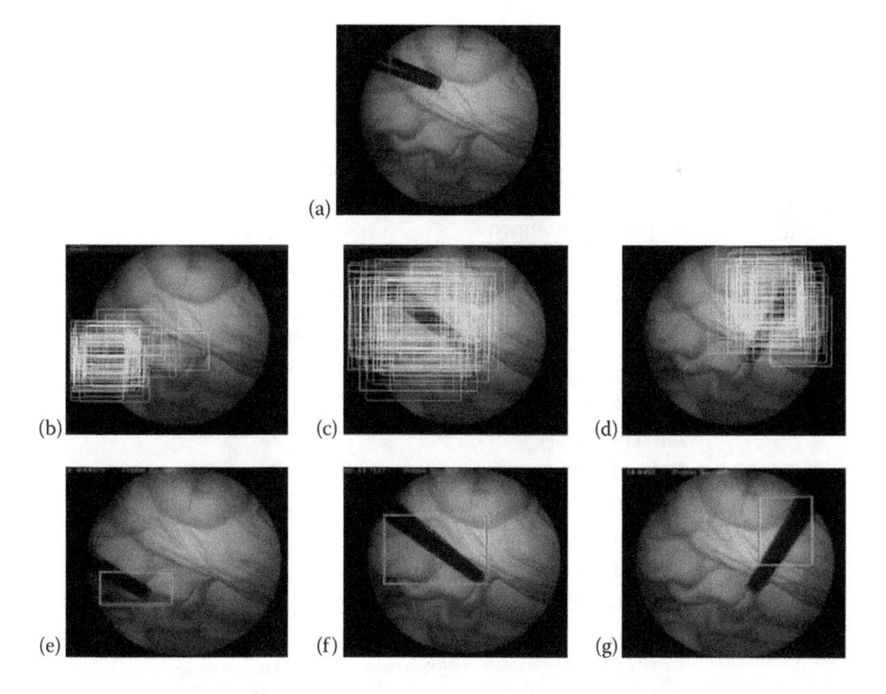

FIGURE 5.8 Tracking results of the modified PF approach in an emulated *in vitro* scene. The initial region is defined in (a); (b), (c), and (d) are the generated particles at different times; (e), (f), and (g) are the tracking results corresponding to (b), (c), and (d).

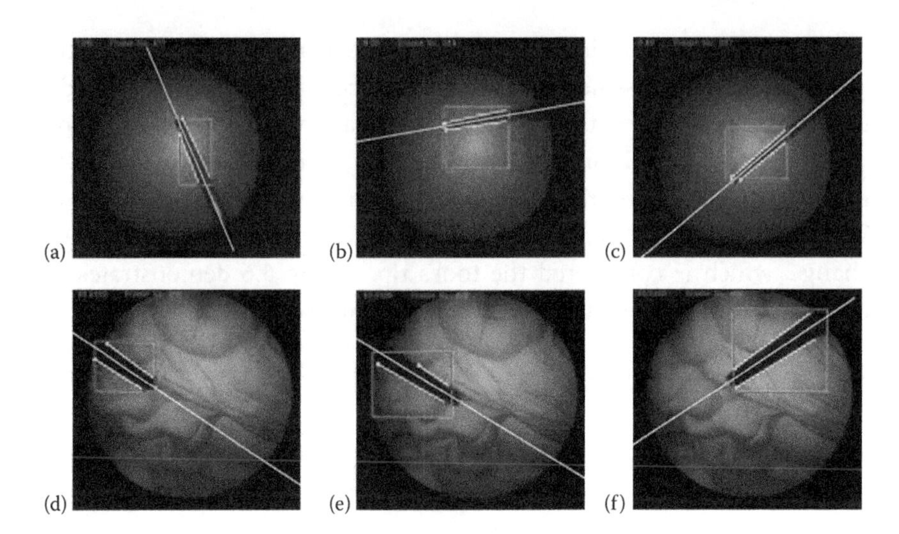

FIGURE 5.9 Tracking results of the hybrid approach in ideal and emulated *in vitro* scenes: (a), (b), and (c) are the results in the ideal scene at different positions; (d), (e), and (f) are the results for the emulated scene.

TABLE 5.1 Tracking Performance of the Modified PF and Hybrid Approaches under Various Real Surgical Environments

	Tracking Success Rate (frames/200 frames *100%)	
Method	**Modified PF (%)**	**Hybrid method (%)**
Ideal scene	80	83
Emulated scene	90	92
Video no. 1	45	20
Video no. 2	50	15
Video no. 3	60	Fail
Video no. 4	67	40
Video no. 5	65	50
Video no. 6	56	17
Video no. 7	58	10
Video no. 8	53	Fail
Video no. 9	Fail	Fail
Video no. 10	15	Fail

For the *in vitro* training experiments, the two methods were tested both in an ideal scene with a clear background and an emulated scene with a complex background. These two types of scenes were captured from the simulated surgical setup. Figures 5.7 and 5.8 are the tracking results of the modified PF method under these two scenes, respectively. The modified PF method requires the user to manually define the initial region using the surgical tool (Figure 5.7a). If the tracking is lost, the user needs to

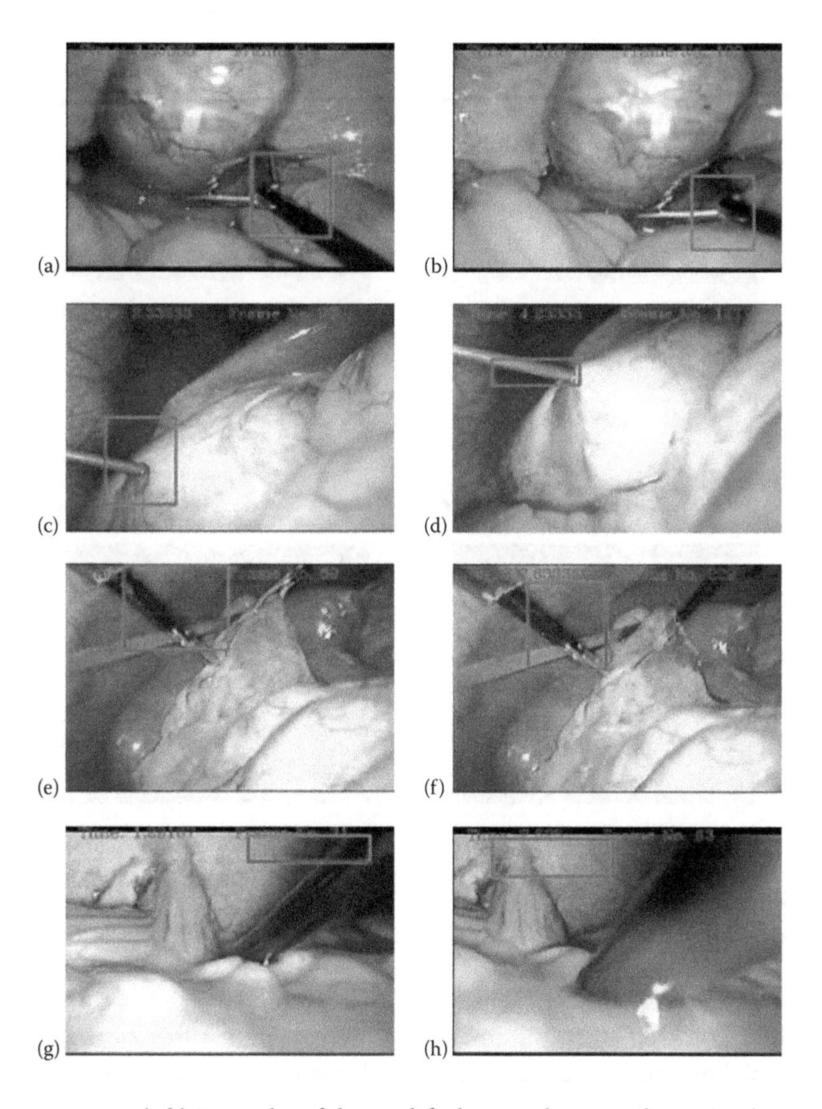

FIGURE 5.10 (a-h) Examples of the modified PF tracking results in a real *in vivo* surgical scene. Rectangles indicate the tracked region from the PF framework.

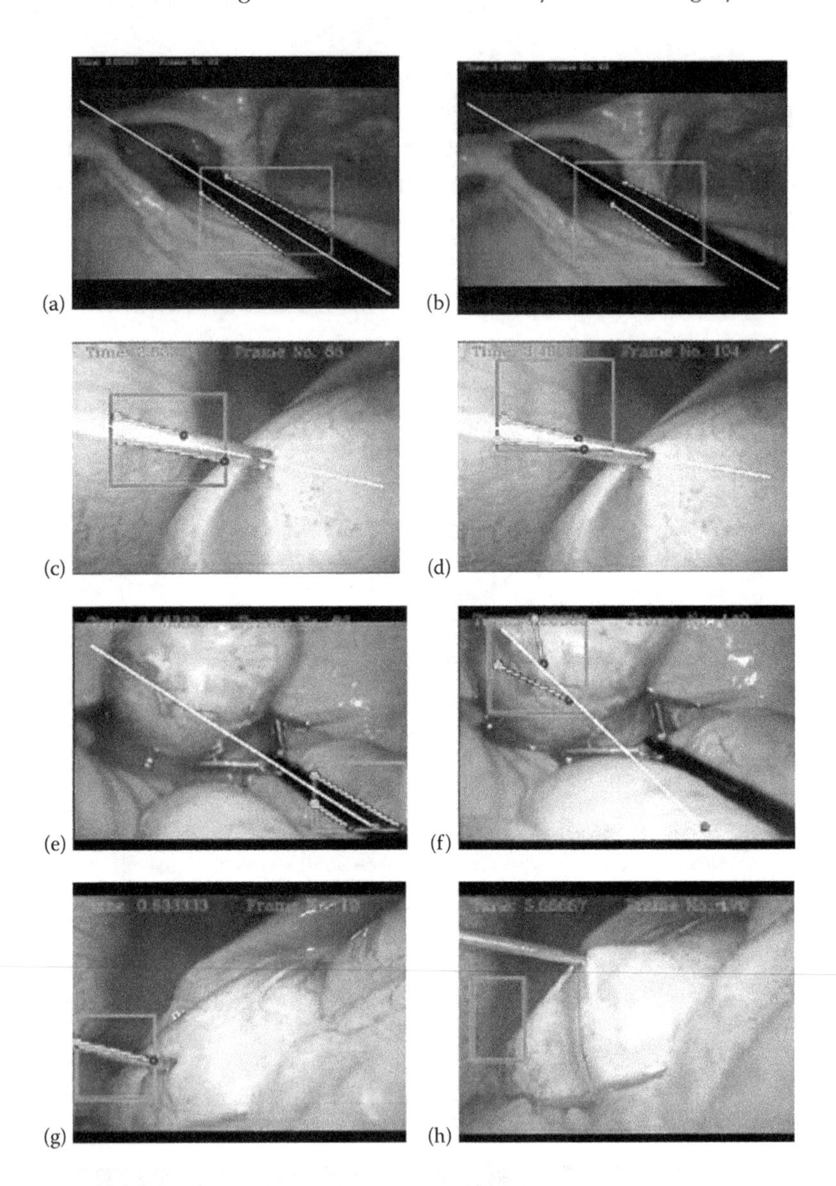

FIGURE 5.11 (a-h) Examples of the hybrid tracking results in a real *in vivo* surgical scene. Rectangles indicate the tracked region from the PF framework; the detected features are indicated within the rectangles.

define the region again to reinitialize the PF framework. For the hybrid method, tracking starts automatically and can return the feature information about the surgical tool. The AGMM can help the PF framework to recover from lost tracking situations. Figure 5.9 demonstrates the *in vitro* tracking results by means of the hybrid method.

To evaluate the tracking performance of these two approaches in an *in vivo* environment and compare the results with the Gaussian-type approaches, we used the same 10 real surgical video streams from the previous chapter for the *in vivo* experiments. The tracking success rates for both methods are listed in Table 5.1. Examples of successful and failed tracking of surgical tools are shown in Figures 5.10 and 5.11.

SUMMARY

In this chapter, three non-Gaussian-type tracking approaches (the PF, modified PF, and hybrid methods) were evaluated for tracking surgical tools in different environments. For the *in vitro* experiment including an ideal scene and an emulated scene, both methods have similar performances in comparison with the Gaussian-type methods presented in the previous chapter. The KF and the EKF methods are sensitive to the background, resulting in a slight decrease in tracking success rates in the emulated scenes. The PF tracking framework can avoid this drawback and even has better performance in the emulated scenes because it relies on the color histogram rather than feature information. For the *in vivo* experiment, the modified PF method has the best tracking results in comparison with all the other methods, even though it fails in some of the more complex surgical scenes and with fast tool motion (Table 5.1). The method is rarely influenced by the color of the tool or its material properties. The color distribution in the user-defined region is distinct from the other areas, so the PF algorithm is able to maintain its accuracy during tracking. As to the hybrid method, it works well in the *in vitro* environment without initialization and is able to come back from lost tracking situations. Moreover, based on the tracked region, it is able to provide information about the features of the tool even if the tracked region covers just a small part of the tool.

CHAPTER 6

Region-Based Tracking

It was shown in the previous chapters that the visual tracking of surgical tools can be used in the implementation of a surgeon–computer interface (SCI). The surgical tools that are being held and manipulated by the surgeon during the training or practice of minimally invasive surgery (MIS) are viewed as a 3-D computer mouse. When needed, medical information and images of the patient can be overlaid on the live image of the surgical site. The surgeon can then use the surgical tools to interact with the overlaid information. For example, it was shown that by using the surgical tools, the surgeon is able to register preoperative images of the patient by manipulating the overlaid images toward the desired location on the surgical scene given an orientation of the endoscope. This further allows the implementation of image-guided surgery using the conventional surgical setup used for MIS.

This chapter explores approaches where anchor points can be created on the live surgical scene, where, regardless of the movements of the endoscope, the overlaid medical images remain anchored in their desired locations. The region-matching procedure is the basis for such augmented enhancement. To highlight some key regions in the surgical scene, the surgeon can mark these regions by manipulating the surgical tool as a 3-D mouse. During the surgery, it is desirable for these marked regions to be identifiable in different scenes caused by changes in the position of the endoscope, illumination, or other viewing conditions. To match the same region in various images, a set of *feature points* to describe the region are identified and then it is distinguished from its surrounding environment. By finding the correspondence between the feature points of two images, we can align the same region in different scenes.

In the following sections, feature-based region-matching methods are introduced, which include the *scale-invariant feature transform* (SIFT), *speeded-up robust features* (SURF), and *oriented FAST and rotated BRIEF* (ORB) algorithms. These methods are first evaluated in general settings in order to evaluate their tracking performance in different viewing conditions, including the *in vitro* emulated surgical scenes. The performances of three of the methods are further evaluated using *in vivo* surgical scenes.

FEATURE DESCRIPTION AND EXTRACTION

Region alignment can play an important role in an SCI system for intraoperative guidance and augmented reality (AR) visualization. Feature-based region alignment is also an approach in image processing and computer vision to deal with image matching and object recognition. This type of approach represents the region of interest as a set of interest points. These points are called *keypoints* or *features*, which are represented using descriptors. A descriptor, just like a human fingerprint, is capable of identifying the same keypoint in different image scenes and is considered the main component of image matching. To extract the discriminative and repeatable features from an image, algorithms such as SIFT (Lowe 2004) and SURF (Bay et al. 2006) have been presented in the last decade. These local features are invariant to different viewing conditions, including image scale, rotation, and illumination change. Recently, more efficient feature-matching methods such as *binary robust independent elementary features* (BRIEF) (Calonder et al. 2010), ORB (Rublee et al. 2011), *binary robust invariant scalable keypoints* (BRISK) (Leutenegger et al. 2011), and *fast retina keypoints* (FREAK) (Alahi et al. 2012) have been proposed to reduce the high computational cost as well as preserving the distinctive property of local features. In the following, three of the above algorithms—namely, the SIFT, SURF, and ORB descriptors—are investigated.

SIFT Description and Extraction

SIFT (Lowe 2004) has been widely used to match features between images from different views. It is able to provide reliable matching when the images have orientation and scale changes owing to its highly discriminating descriptor. The four major stages of the SIFT algorithm include building Gaussian scale space, detecting and locating keypoints, assigning reference orientations to keypoints, and finally producing a keypoint descriptor.

To find the stable features that are invariant to image scale change under different viewing conditions of the same region, a scale space is created using a set of Gaussian kernels $G_{x,\,y}(\sigma)$ with variant scale σ. Here it is assumed that the input image has the intensity $I_{x,\,y}$ at the pixel location (x, y). The scale space $L_{x,\,y}(\sigma)$ is then defined as the convolution of the image and Gaussian function as $L_{x,\,y}(\sigma) = G_{x,\,y}(\sigma) * I_{x,\,y}$.

The notion of *octave* is then introduced to classify the scale space according to image resolution. Images with the same octave have the same resolution but they are convoluted by different Gaussian kernels with various scales. The pyramid structure is applied to produce multilevel scale space where the new octave is generated by down-sampling the original input image.

Figure 6.1 illustrates an example of a Gaussian scale space with four octaves and five scales. The original 512×512 image is resampled three times to produce the input images for the second, third, and fourth octaves. These images are smoothed by five Gaussian kernels with different scales.

To find the keypoint candidates in this scale space, we need to generate a set of difference-of-Gaussian (DoG) images by subtracting adjacent Gaussian images in each octave.

As shown in Figure 6.2, the maxima and minima of the DoG image sets are detected by comparing the current pixel with its 26 surrounding neighbors. These neighbors are from the current octave and two nearby octaves as well. The detected keypoint candidates may contain interfering points that have low contrast or are poorly determined along the edge, so that a filtering step is required to eliminate these points.

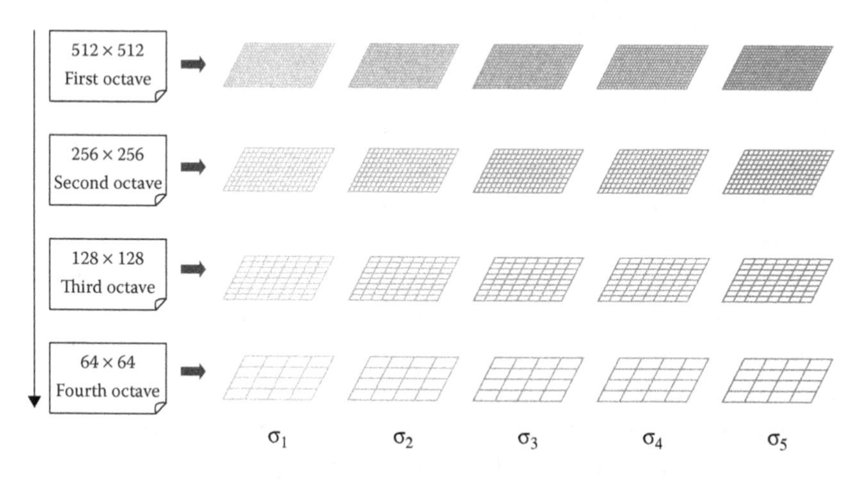

FIGURE 6.1 Visualization of Gaussian scale space with four octaves and five scales.

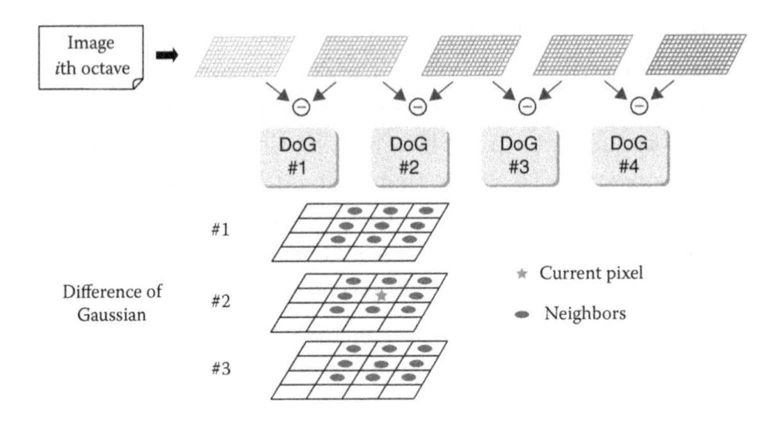

FIGURE 6.2 Formation of DoG images at the *i*th octave and the definition of the 26 surrounding neighbors.

To make the keypoint descriptor invariant to image rotation, a consistent orientation needs to be assigned to each detected keypoint based on the local image properties around it. Given the smoothed Gaussian image $L_{x,y}$ at scale σ, the gradient magnitude is defined as

$$M_{x,y} = \sqrt{\left(L_{x+1,y} - L_{x-1,y}\right)^2 + \left(L_{x,y+1} - L_{x,y-1}\right)^2}$$

and the direction at location (x, y) is computed as $\theta_{x,y} = \tan^{-1}[(L_{x,y+1} - L_{x,y-1})/(L_{x+1,y} - L_{x-1,y})]$.

For each keypoint, we consider all the sample points within the local region around the keypoint. The gradient orientations of these sample points are weighted by their gradient magnitudes and a Gaussian-weighted circular window with 1.5σ. By analyzing the orientation distribution of these sample points, we can assign a dominant orientation to the keypoint and further create new keypoints sharing the same location (x, y) and scale σ but which have various orientations.

Given the location, scale, and orientation for each keypoint, the descriptor is then designed to distinguish one keypoint from another. For example, a 128-element feature vector can be used to describe a keypoint. This vector is created from the 16×16 sample array around each keypoint containing both the orientation and magnitude information in the local region (Appendix IV). By comparing the SIFT descriptors in two images, we are able to find the corresponding feature points between them. Figures 6.3 and 6.4 give two examples of extracted feature points using the SIFT algorithm in a general scene and a surgical scene.

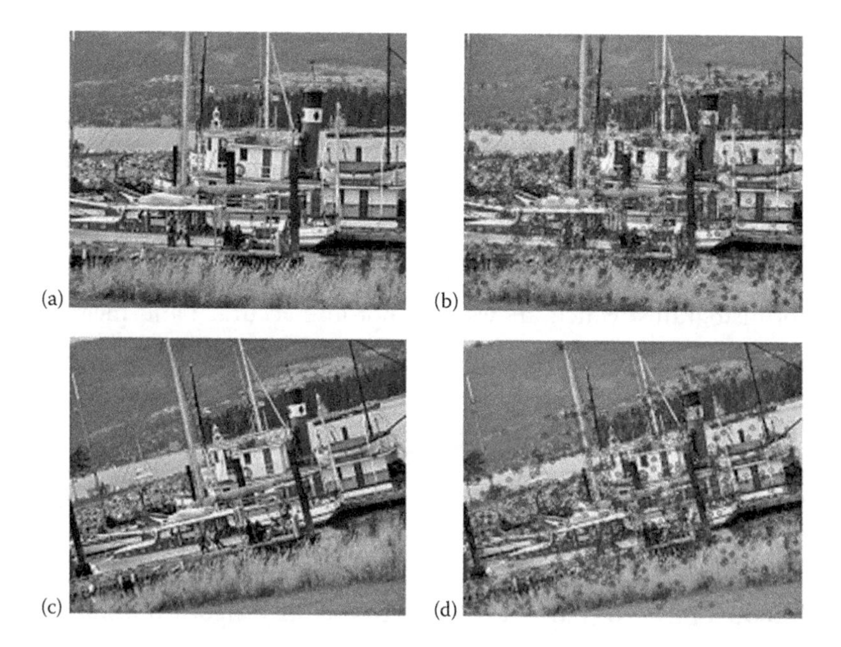

FIGURE 6.3 SIFT feature detection in two images with different views: (a) and (c) are the two boat images from the Oxford dataset; (c) has a slight rotation compared with (a); (b) and (d) are the results after SIFT feature detection, where circles indicate the detected features.

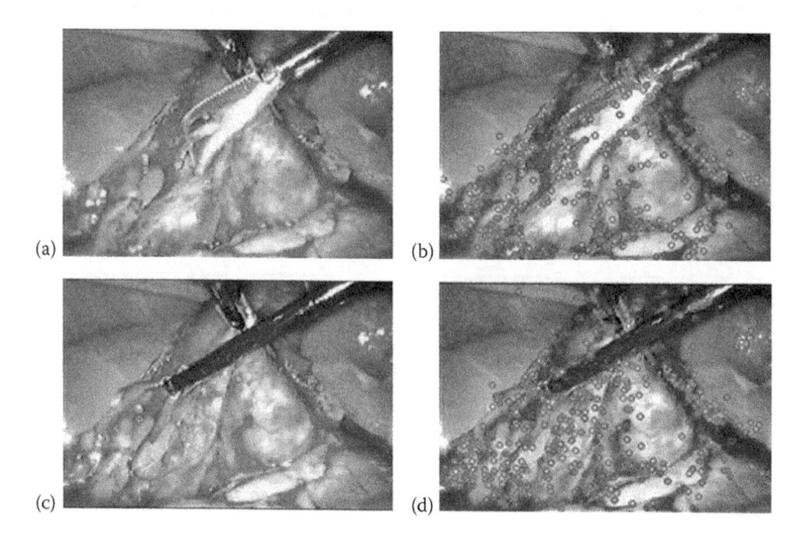

FIGURE 6.4 SIFT feature detection in two surgical scenes: (a) and (c) are two different moments during laparoscopic surgery (the data are from the video clip); (b) and (d) are the results after SIFT feature detection, where circles indicate the detected features.

SURF Description and Extraction

Although the SIFT method provides repeatability and distinctiveness for feature matching, it has an increased computational cost due to the high dimensionality of the descriptor. There are many other approaches proposed in the literature to solve this problem, among which the SURF detector-descriptor scheme is one of the most popular (Bay et al. 2006). Similar to the SIFT method, the SURF scheme relies on the local gradient of histograms, which allows it to not lose accuracy and meanwhile takes advantage of integral images to reduce the running time (Viola and Jones 2001).

The feature detection step in the SURF scheme is based on a fast-Hessian detector. The second-order Gaussian derivatives are replaced by box filters that can be quickly evaluated using integral images, independently of size. For instance, a 9×9 box filter can approximate the second-order Gaussian derivatives with scale $\sigma=1.2$, and a 27×27 box filter corresponds to one with $\sigma=3\times1.2=3.6$ (Bay et al. 2006). In the SIFT algorithm, the image pyramid is generated by resampling the image size. In the SURF scheme, the scale space is organized by scaling the filter size and applying these filters to the original input image. The big mask can create not only higher image levels but also new octaves in the pyramid. Figure 6.5 demonstrates the SURF scale space with four octaves and three levels. Specifically, the size of the mask is doubled in the nearby upper octave, such as from 6 to 12 to 24. To detect the keypoint, a *nonmaximum suppression* is applied in a $3\times3\times3$ neighborhood in each octave across adjacent levels (Figure 6.5).

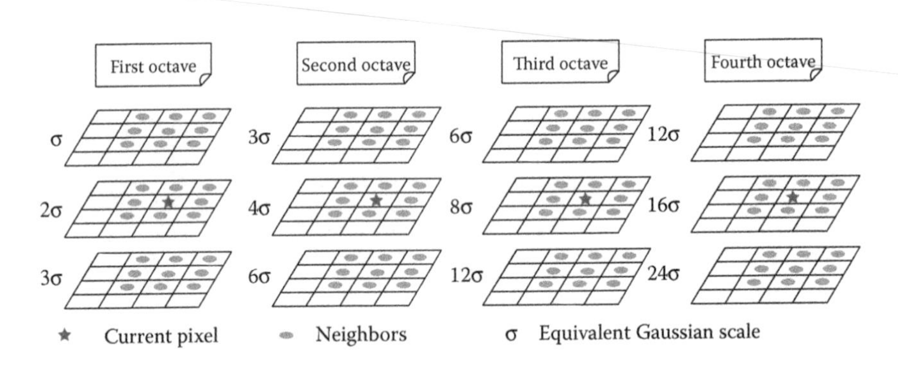

FIGURE 6.5 Example of the SURF scale space with four octaves and three levels. The $3\times3\times3$ neighborhood is shown for each octave. For each level, the size of the filter is represented in the form of its equivalent Gaussian scale. A 9×9 box filter can approximate the second-order derivatives with scale $\sigma=1.2$.

(Nonmaximum suppression is an edge-thinning technique originally from Canny detection. Every pixel is compared with its neighbors; if the magnitude of the center point is greater than the magnitude of its neighbors, the center point is kept, otherwise it is set to zero.) To further overcome the huge scale difference between the first layers of adjacent octaves, the scale space interpolation method is applied (Brown and Lowe 2002).

The SURF descriptor is constructed based on similar local image properties in the SIFT descriptor but is more efficient using integral images. The scale and the location of the keypoint is determined by the Hessian matrix. The reproducible orientation of the keypoint is computed from the Haar wavelet responses. Based on the information of scale, location, and orientation, a 64-dimension descriptor vector is assigned to each keypoint. An alternative version called SURF-128 extends the number of descriptor entries to 128 by introducing similar features (Appendix IV). The extracted feature points using the SURF algorithm in a general scene and a surgical scene are displayed in Figures 6.6 and 6.7, respectively.

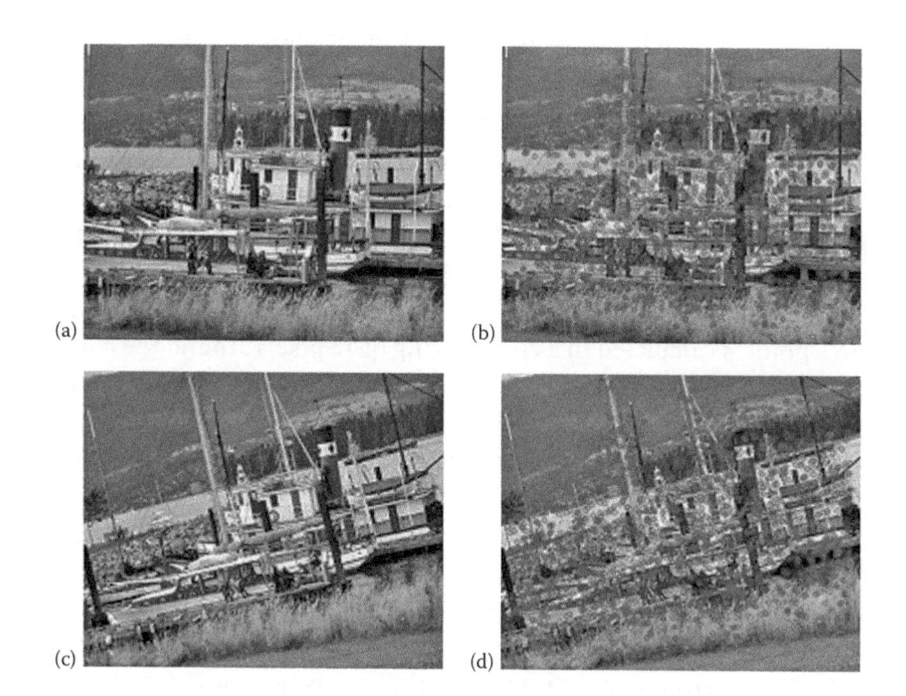

FIGURE 6.6 SURF feature detection in two boat images with different views: (a) and (c) are the same two input images as those in Figure 6.3; (b) and (d) are the results after SURF feature detection, where circles indicate the detected features.

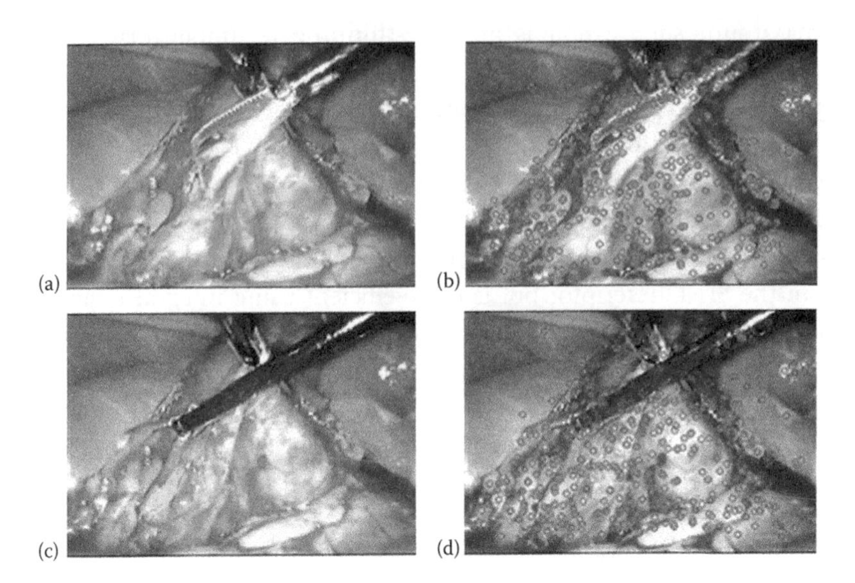

FIGURE 6.7 SURF feature detection in two surgical scenes: (a) and (c) are the same two input images as those in Figure 6.4; (b) and (d) are the results after SURF feature detection, where circles indicate the detected features.

ORB Description and Extraction

A more computationally efficient approach was presented recently aiming at extending the feature detection and matching into real-time applications (Rublee et al. 2011). This approach is based on both the *features from accelerated segment test* (FAST) corner detector (Rosten and Drummond 2006) and the BRIEF descriptor (Calonder et al. 2010). The FAST point is calculated in a circular ring of 16 pixels around the corner candidate p (Figure 6.8). An intensity threshold is set to test whether there exists n contiguous pixels within the circular region all brighter or darker than p. As long as either of these two cases happens, p is considered a corner.

In the ORB algorithm, n is chosen as 9, which performs well. To reject edges and provide a reasonable score, the Harris corner filter is applied to order the detected FAST keypoints. Moreover, an image scale pyramid is also added to produce multiscale features. Since the FAST detector does not contain orientation information, the intensity centroid technique (Rosin 1999) is used to assign the single dominant direction to each FAST keypoint. To improve the rotation invariance, the centroid technique is limited to a circular region of radius r, known as the *patch size*.

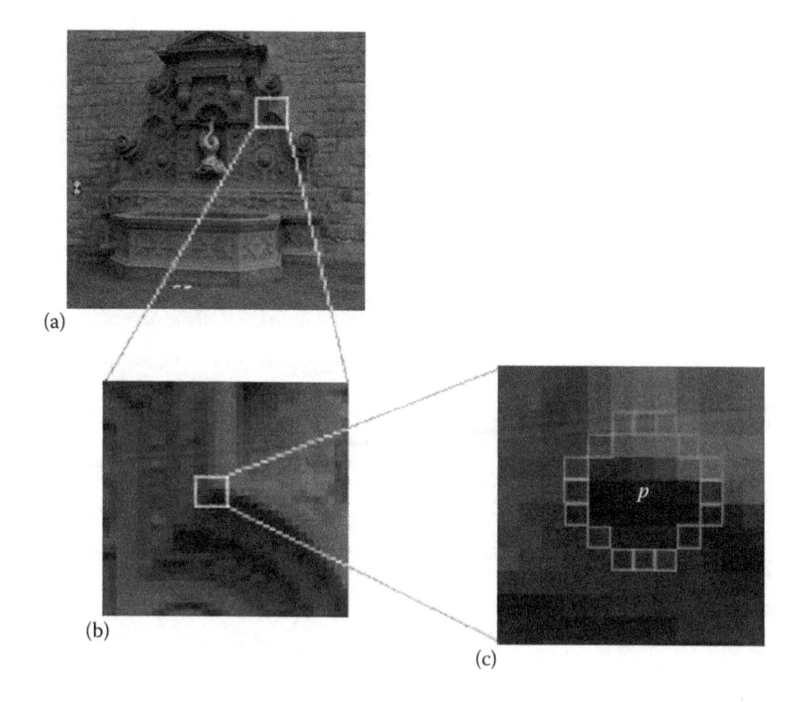

FIGURE 6.8 FAST corner test within a circular ring area around the candidate point p: (a) is the original fountain image; (b) is the corner part we want to detect. In (c), the 16 surrounding points indicated by squares are compared with a threshold to see whether they can form a contiguous segment.

The BRIEF descriptor is created from a set of binary intensity tests with a smoothed image patch (Calonder et al. 2010). The binary test τ is defined as

$$\tau(p;x,y)=\begin{cases}1 & \text{if } p(x)<p(y)\\ 0 & \text{otherwise}\end{cases} \tag{6.1}$$

where $p(x)$ is the intensity value of image patch p at pixel x. Assuming we have n number of (x, y) location pairs, the feature descriptor is an n-dimensional bit string expressed as

$$f_n(p)=\sum_{1\le i\le n} 2^{i-1}\tau(p;x_i,y_i) \tag{6.2}$$

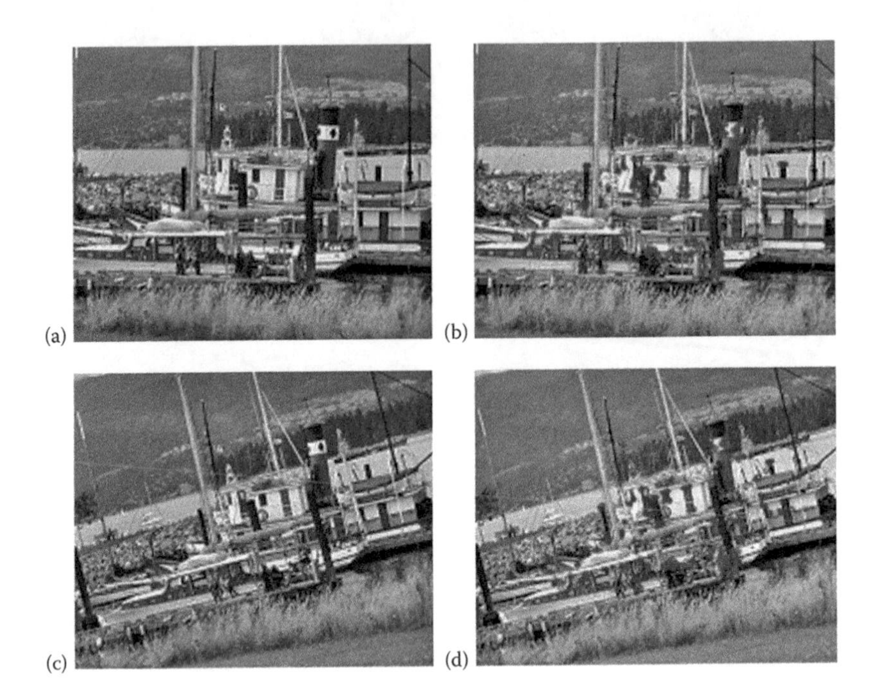

FIGURE 6.9 ORB feature detection in two boat images with different views: (a) and (c) are the same two input images as those in Figure 6.3; (b) and (d) are the results after ORB feature detection, where circles indicate the detected features.

In the ORB algorithm, n is set to 256. To allow the BRIEF descriptor to be invariant to in-plane rotation, the original descriptor is steered according to the orientation of the keypoints (Appendix IV). To keep high variance and uncorrelation among the binary tests, a learning method is utilized for optimizing the binary tests, such as a *greedy search* (Rublee et al. 2011). Examples of ORB detection in a general case and a surgical case are shown in Figures 6.9 and 6.10, respectively.

MEASURING FEATURE MATCHING

Using the descriptors defined in the previous section, the image now contains a number of feature points that uniquely indicate various regions. To match the same region under different camera views, we need to know the corresponding relationship between the features in two images. Since the feature descriptors are represented as multidimensional vectors, the distance between vectors is considered the matching criterion. To find the best match between two sets of features, numerous descriptor matchers

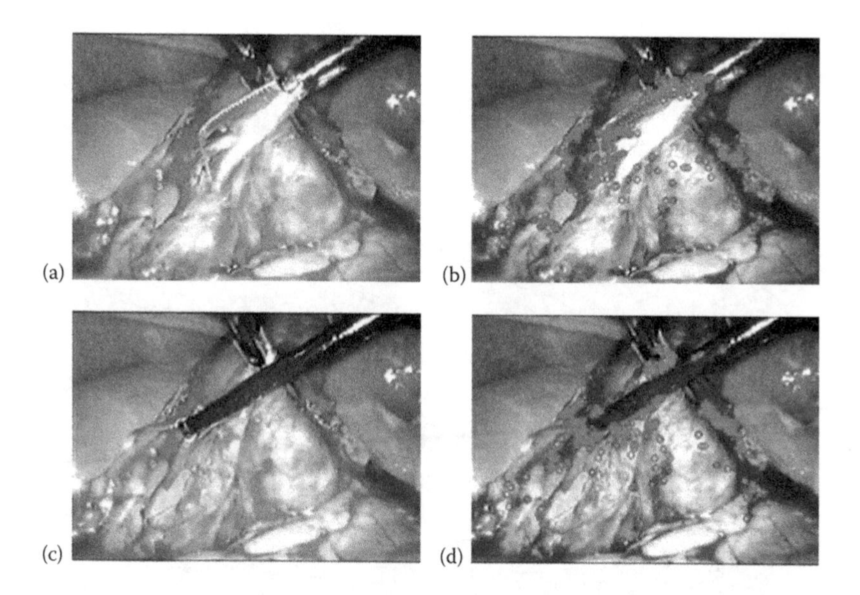

FIGURE 6.10 ORB feature detection in two surgical scenes: (a) and (c) are the same two input images as those in Figure 6.4; (b) and (d) are the results after ORB feature detection, where circles indicate the detected features.

have been proposed in recent decades. Particularly, the *brute-force* (BF) matcher and the *fast library for approximate nearest neighbors* (FLANN) (Muja and Lowe 2009) matcher are the most popular. In the experimental study of this chapter, the BF matcher is selected due to its simplicity and acceptable practical performance.

The BF matcher is a simple searching algorithm that enumerates all of the possible candidates in the second set and finds the closest one compared with the object in the first set according to certain distance measurements from each of the candidates. The L_1 and L_2 distances are usually the choices for the SIFT and the SURF descriptors. Given two descriptor vectors, $U=(u_1, u_2, \ldots, u_n)$ and $V=(v_1, v_2, \ldots, v_n)$, their L_1 distance is $L_1(U,V)=\sum_{i=1}^{n} u_i - v_i$ and their L_2 distance is $L_2(U,V)=\sum_{i=1}^{n}(u_i - v_i)^2$. For the ORB descriptor, the Hamming distance is used to evaluate the difference between two binary strings. It returns the number of corresponding positions with different entries, which can be expressed as

$$L_{\text{Hamming}} = \sum_{i=1}^{n} XOR(u_i, v_i) \tag{6.3}$$

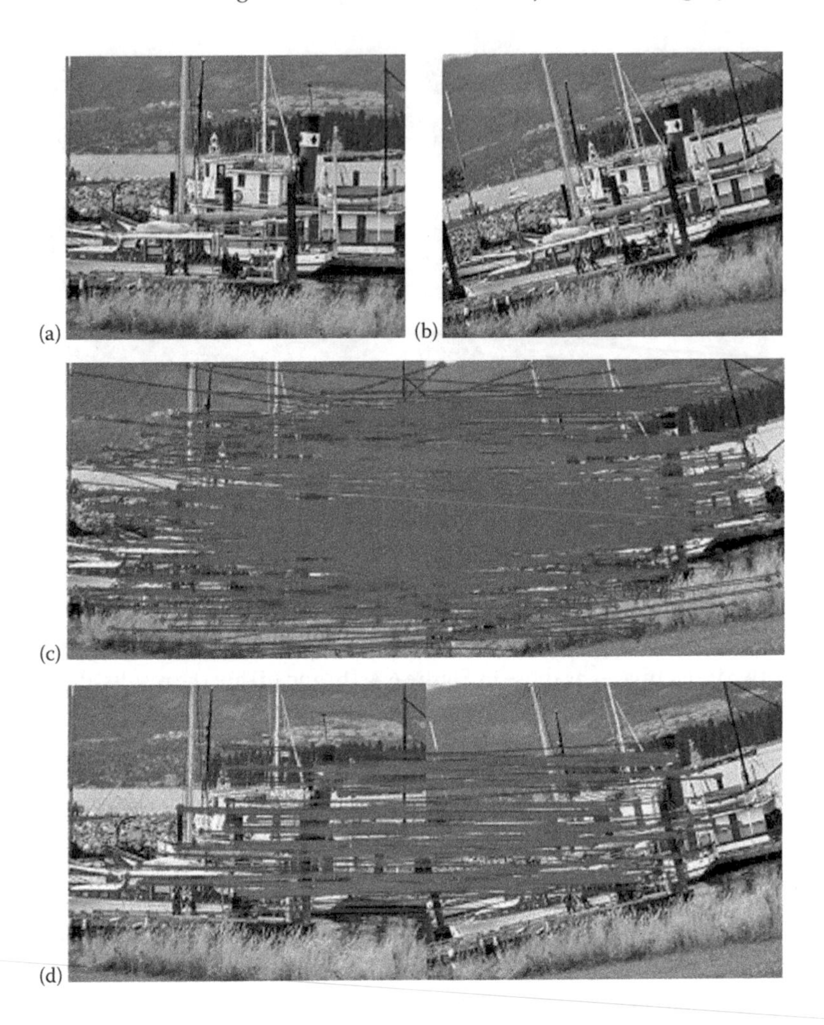

FIGURE 6.11 Feature matching using the BF matcher for a general scene: (a) and (b) are the input boat images; (c) and (d) are the feature matching results for SIFT and ORB descriptors, respectively. In (c), the $L2$ distances between SIFT features are selected as the measurement, while in (d), the Hamming distances are calculated between two ORB descriptors.

Given two descriptor sets $S[n_s]$ and $T[n_t]$, we want to use the BF searching algorithm to find the closest match for each member in the set $S[n_s]$. D_{dist} is the selected distance measurement and the minimum distance is labeled as D_{min}. The matching results are stored in the descriptor set $M[n_s]$.

Figures 6.11 and 6.12 demonstrate the matching results based on the BF searching algorithm. A distance threshold is set to remove outliers among the matching pairs, keeping only the ones with a low calculated distance.

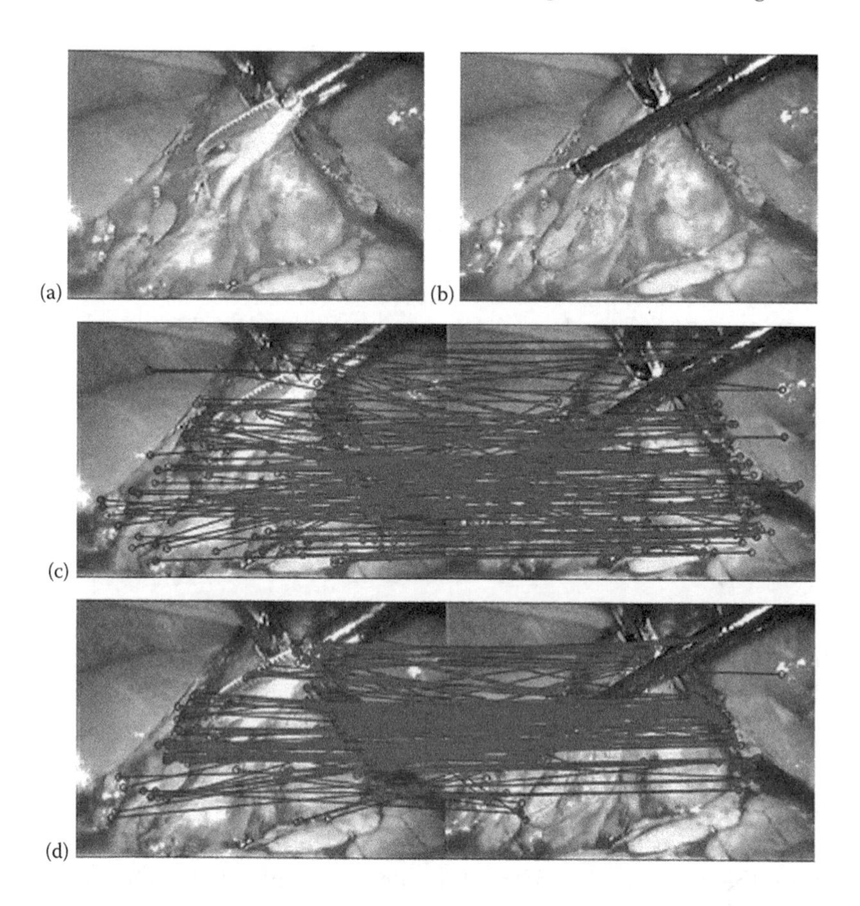

FIGURE 6.12 Feature matching using the BF matcher for surgical scene: (a) and (b) are the input laparoscopic images; (c) and (d) are the feature matching results for SURF and ORB descriptors, respectively. In (c), the $L2$ distances between SURF features are selected as the measurement, while in (d), the Hamming distances are calculated between two ORB descriptors.

ESTIMATION OF PLANAR HOMOGRAPHY

From the feature pairs we have found using the descriptor-matching algorithm, the objective is to indicate the same object under different views using geometrical transformation. Planar homography, defined as projective mapping from one plane to another, can be used to analytically express such transformations as a 3×3 matrix (Hartley and Zisserman 2006) (Figure 6.13). Given two planes S and T, which represent the source and target planes, respectively, the mapping between the points on these two planes can be expressed in terms of matrix multiplication:

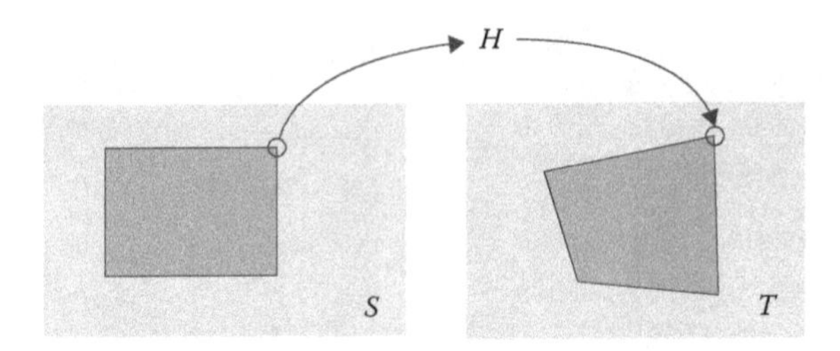

FIGURE 6.13 The planar homography transformation H defines the mapping from plane S to plane T. The corresponding points are indicated by circles.

$$\begin{bmatrix} x_T \\ y_T \\ 1 \end{bmatrix} = H \begin{bmatrix} x_S \\ y_S \\ 1 \end{bmatrix} \tag{6.4}$$

where $[x, y, 1]^T$ is the homogeneous coordinates of the points.

From a list of corresponding points, the homography matrix H can be computed based on all the input point pairs using a simple least squares scheme. However, this method is sensitive to outliers if not all the point pairs fit the transformation. An alternative method called the *random sample consensus* (RANSAC) algorithm (Appendix IV) is capable of estimating the homography matrix (Fischler and Bolles 1981). On the basis of the assumption that the input data consist of *inliers* and few *outliers*, RANSAC makes use of a small set of data points to estimate the initial mathematical model and iteratively improve the model by adding consistent data points into the set.

To highlight the target region in the image, a novel user-friendly interaction step is designed and implemented to allow the user to define the region they want to match. Figure 6.14 displays several examples of region definition. Using a mouse as a computer interface device and a surgical tool as a 3-D mouse, the user can select several positions (i.e., green points) as the vertexes of a region polygon. This region polygon is also applied to generate a mask when doing the feature description and extraction so that only the features within the region polygon are calculated and matched. The tool's tip position is sent to the computer by the visual tracking module so that the user can define the region using their surgical tool. In accordance with

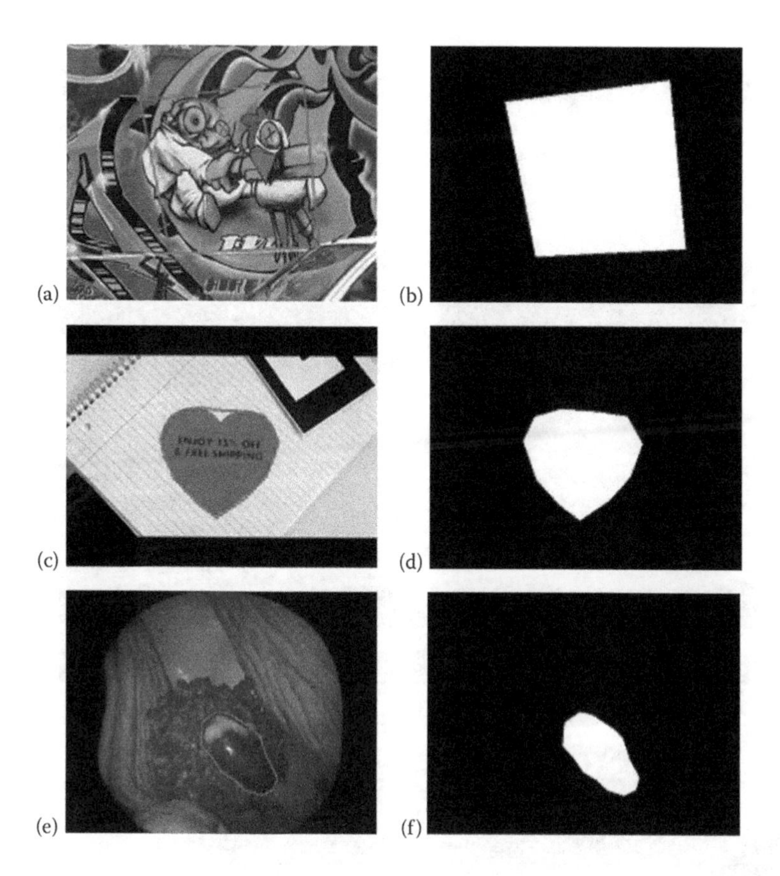

FIGURE 6.14 Region selection and mask generation: (a) and (c) are the general images from the Oxford dataset and our lab, respectively; (e) is captured from the endoscope setup in our lab. The areas highlighted by the polygons in the first column are the regions selected by the user. The second column (b,d, and f) shows the accordingly generated masks that will be applied in feature matching.

the estimated homography matrix and Equation 6.4, the transformed region polygon can be computed as

$$V_{dst} = HV_{scr} \tag{6.5}$$

where V represents the vertexes of the region polygon. Figures 6.15 and 6.16 give examples of how we match regions in different views by matching the features in the region. The user is first allowed to select the region

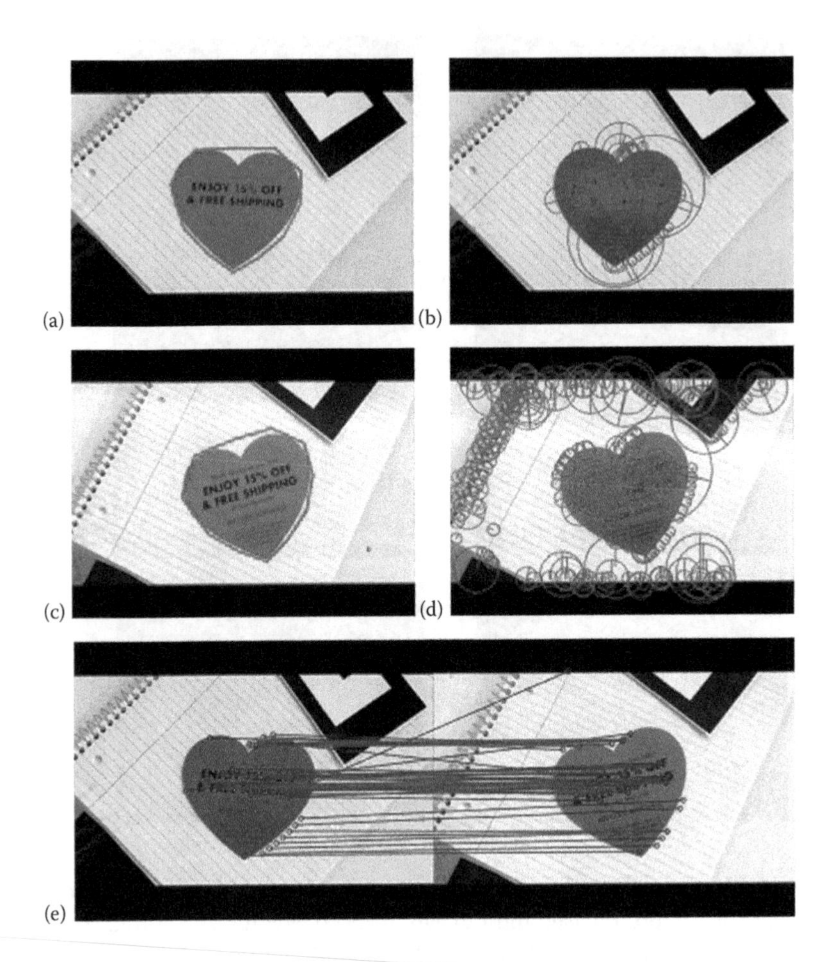

FIGURE 6.15 Region matching based on the SURF descriptor. The polygon indicates the selected region in the source image (a). The SURF feature descriptors within the region are shown in (b) by circles. Similar to those in (d), the size and direction of the circles refer to the magnitude and orientation of the descriptors. The matched region in (c) is obtained according to the homography matrix, which is calculated from the corresponding features in (e).

of interest using the mouse, and a region mask is generated accordingly. By applying the mask to the source image, we only need to calculate the local features within the mask. These features are compared with the features over the entire destination image. The well-matched feature points are connected by the blue lines (Figures 6.15e and 6.16e). The homography matrix is computed from these well-matched feature points and is applied to obtain the transformed region polygon.

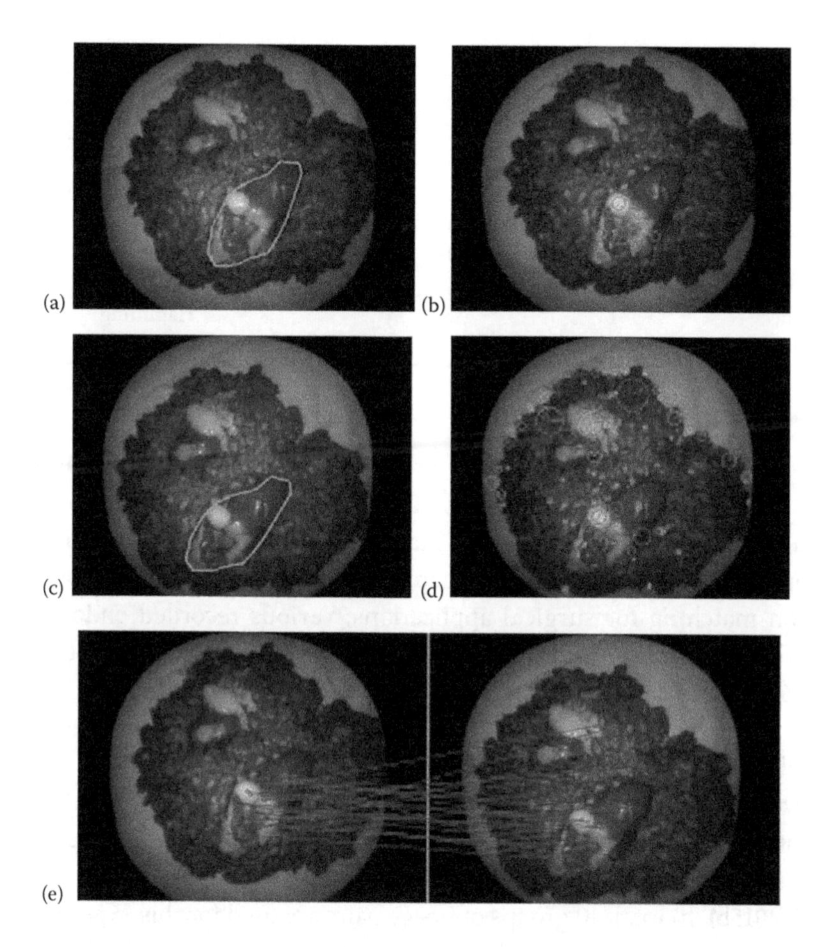

FIGURE 6.16 Region matching example in an emulated surgical scene based on the SIFT descriptor. The polygon indicates the selected region in the source image (a). The SIFT feature descriptors within the region are shown in (b) by red circles. Similar to those in (d), the size and direction of the circles refer to the magnitude and orientation of the descriptors. The matched region in (c) is obtained according to the homography matrix, which is calculated from the corresponding features in (e).

EXPERIMENTAL STUDIES

In this section, feature-based region matching is experimentally studied using image data and video data from a general environment, an emulated environment, and a surgical environment. To test the SIFT, SURF, and ORB feature detection algorithms in the general case, we use data from the Oxford dataset [44], the Strecha dataset [45], the Heinly dataset [46],

TABLE 6.1 Parameter Setting for SIFT, SURF, and ORB Descriptors

Descriptor	SIFT	SURF	ORB
Parameter setting	Number of octaves is autocomputed from image resolution Number of levels is four	Number of octaves is three Number of levels is four 128-element descriptor	Number of features is 500 Score type is Harris score
Distance measurement	L_2	L_2	Hamming

and our laboratory. Before we extend the experimental study to cases of real MIS scenes, some emulated matching tests are first conducted. The data for this part of the study are obtained from the *in vitro* experimental setup presented in the previous chapters. For evaluation of the proposed region matching for surgical applications, various recorded endoscopic videos of actual surgical scenes are used. For all of the above studies, Table 6.1 defines the parameters that were used in each of the algorithms.

Testing Results of General Image Data

To evaluate the performance of the SIFT, SURF, and ORB methods under different viewing conditions, such as viewpoint change, rotation, and blurring, we first test the feature matching over the entire image (Zhou 2014; Zhou et al. 2015b). In total, 10 groups of image pairs are used for this experiment. Seven of them are from well-known datasets: *Bikes*, *Leuven*, *Graffiti*, *Boat* (Mikolajczyk et al. 2005), *Fountain* (Strecha et al. 2008), *Venice*, and *Ceiling* (Heinly et al. 2012). The other three are from our lab: *Book*, *U-Pass*, and *Heart Shape*. These image pairs involve different viewing conditions such as blurring (*Bikes*), exposure (*Leuven*), viewpoint change (*Graffiti*, *Fountain*), rotation (*Ceiling*, *Boat*), zooming in (*Venice*), and general transformation (*Book*, *Heart Shape*, and *U-Pass*). To reduce redundancy, the matched feature pairs are further filtered, and we only keep those that have a short distance in the selected feature space, associated parameters setting and the distance measured defined in Table 6.1 (shorter than the average). These feature pairs are called *well-matched pairs*. The accuracy of matching is related to the number of features detected and the similarity of two corresponding features. Table 6.2 lists the number of detected features for each case.

To validate the similarity of two features, we compute the distance between every pair of corresponding feature points and analyze their

TABLE 6.2 Number of Features of SIFT, SURF, and ORB Methods in General Scene Testing

		Number of Features		
Group	**Image Size**	**SIFT**	**SURF**	**ORB**
Bikes	480×336	587	569	500
Leuven	480×320	567	694	488
Graffiti	480×384	927	1698	500
Fountain	480×320	374	456	470
Venice	480×360	897	1133	500
Boat	480×384	1564	2114	500
Ceiling	480×640	4653	2881	500
Book	640×360	524	697	500
U-Pass	640×360	235	401	498
Heart Shape	458×344	251	325	450

distribution. Due to the particularity of each descriptor, they require various distance measurements. As a result, the normalization procedure is necessary before we do the comparison. The linear normalization for a given distance $d_i \epsilon D$ is

$$d_i^* = \frac{d_i - d_{\min}}{d_{\max} - d_{\min}}$$

where $d_{\min}$ is the minimum value and $d_{\min}$ is the maximum value in the distance set D.

Equation 6.6 gives the definition of the standard deviation of the normalized distance D^*:

$$S(D^*) = \sqrt{\frac{\sum (d_i^* - \bar{d}^*)^2}{N}} \tag{6.6}$$

where $\bar{d}^*$ is the average value of D^*. The normalized mean value and standard deviation for the three algorithms are shown in Table 6.3 and Figure 6.17.

The computational cost for each algorithm is compared under different image sizes. Given two image pairs, we resample them into various image sizes and test the SIFT, SURF, and ORB algorithms on the resized images.

TABLE 6.3 Normalized Mean Value and Standard Deviation of SIFT, SURF, and ORB Methods in General Scene Testing

	SIFT			SURF			ORB		
Group	**Time(s)**	**Mean**	**STD**	**Time(s)**	**Mean**	**STD**	**Time(s)**	**Mean**	**STD**
Bikes	1.90	0.67	0.22	1.25	0.39	0.19	0.19	0.48	0.24
Leuven	1.93	0.51	0.28	1.20	0.40	0.23	0.15	0.47	0.25
Graffiti	3.04	0.50	0.27	2.44	0.43	0.18	0.17	0.47	0.24
Fountain	1.71	0.61	0.22	0.73	0.48	0.16	0.12	0.53	0.16
Venice	3.19	0.55	0.30	0.79	0.48	0.20	0.17	0.67	0.20
Boat	4.07	0.54	0.28	3.10	0.43	0.16	0.2	0.47	0.21
Ceiling	12.9	0.41	0.28	4.58	0.47	0.16	0.3	0.46	0.27
Book	2.55	0.45	0.25	1.65	0.44	0.21	0.14	0.56	0.22
U-Pass	2.32	0.51	0.27	0.92	0.42	0.22	0.11	0.52	0.18
Heart Shape	1.48	0.42	0.24	0.72	0.28	0.22	0.18	0.50	0.22

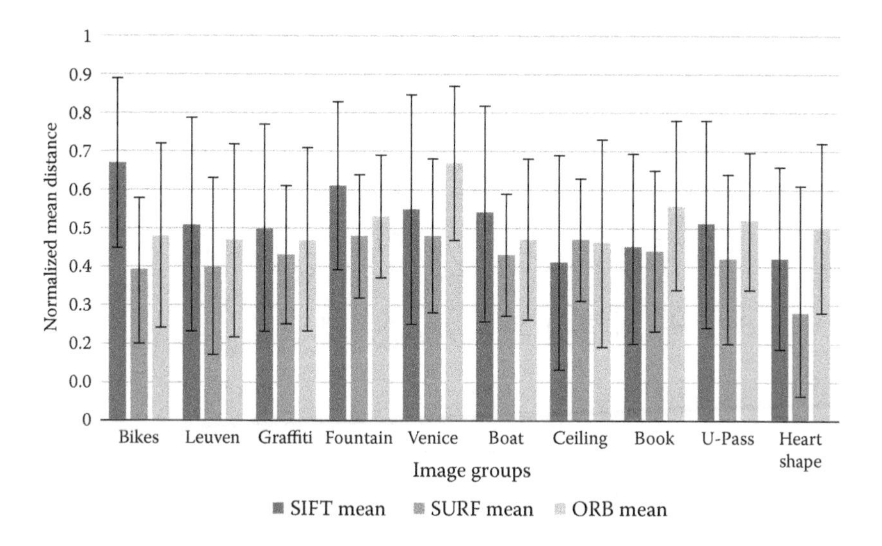

FIGURE 6.17 Normalized mean value and standard deviation for SIFT, SURF, and ORB matching different image groups.

Figure 6.18 illustrates the computational cost for the three methods to match the *Graffiti* image pairs in various sizes.

For region matching, a user-defined mask is necessary to highlight specific regions in the source image. Table 6.4 shows the normalized mean value, standard deviation, and computational cost for the three methods when we use a region mask to shrink the number of features in the source image. Figure 6.19 demonstrates part of the SIFT tracking results when the mask is used. The polygon indicates the same region under different

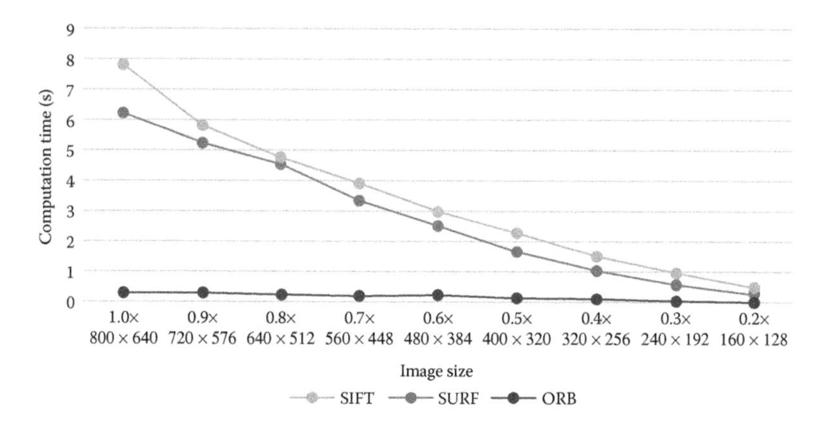

FIGURE 6.18 Cost of computation for SIFT, SURF, and ORB for different size images.

TABLE 6.4 Normalized Mean Value, Standard Deviation, and Computational Costs of All Three Methods Using the Region-Masking Approach

	SIFT			SURF			ORB		
Group	**Time(s)**	**Mean**	**STD**	**Time(s)**	**Mean**	**STD**	**Time(s)**	**Mean**	**STD**
Bikes	1.54	0.73	0.24	0.70	0.44	0.23	0.11	0.67	0.16
Leuven	1.56	0.58	0.28	0.61	0.47	0.28	0.17	0.47	0.25
Graffiti	2.53	0.47	0.3	1.95	0.45	0.18	0.2	0.47	0.25
Fountain	1.46	0.58	0.26	0.44	0.39	0.27	0.18	0.53	0.16
Venice	2.21	0.34	0.36	0.99	0.34	0.34	0.12	0.63	0.26
Boat	3.0	0.51	0.30	1.49	0.44	0.19	0.19	0.59	0.20
Ceiling	7.44	0.36	0.28	2.78	0.51	0.18	0.28	0.48	0.29
Book	2.33	0.37	0.25	1.22	0.42	0.2	0.16	0.56	0.22
U-Pass	1.91	0.39	0.29	0.75	0.42	0.22	0.14	0.45	0.23
Heart Shape	1.52	0.32	0.24	0.40	0.38	0.17	0.13	0.5	0.22

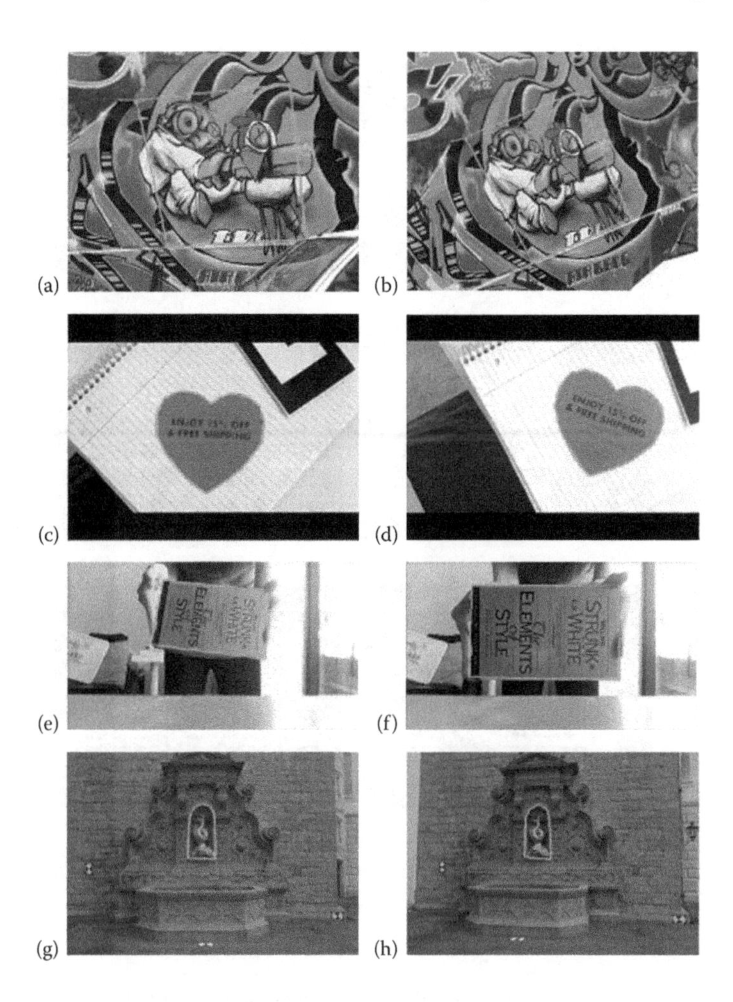

FIGURE 6.19 Examples of SIFT region-matching results using a mask. The left column is the source image and the right column is the target image. The polygon indicates the same region under different viewing conditions, including viewpoint change (a,b and g,h), object planar motion (c,d), and zooming in (e,f). All three methods have similar tracking results dealing with these cases.

viewing conditions, including viewpoint change (Figure 6.19a,b and g,h), object planar motion (Figure 6.19c,d), and zooming in (Figure 6.19e,f). All three methods have similar tracking results dealing with these cases.

The input image pairs for the emulated environment test are classified into two sets: ones with a clean background and ones with a complex background. All the images used in this section have the resolution 640×480. To simplify the experiment, we fix the illumination and ignore the blurring effect. Moreover, considering the specificity of the endoscope, we limit both the motion of the

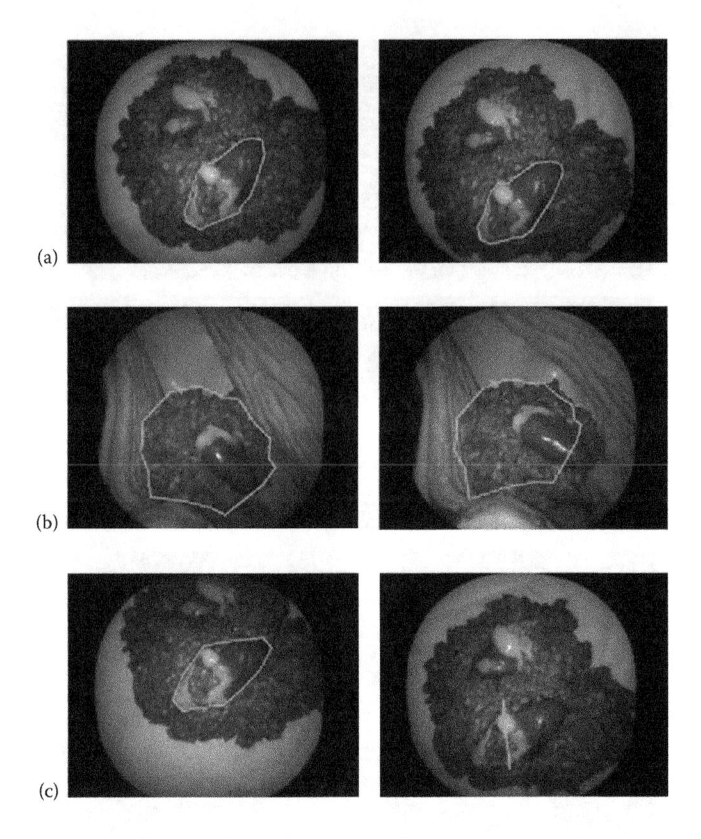

FIGURE 6.20 Description of three region-matching results. (a) GOOD; (b) OK; (c) FAIL.

object and the camera, resulting in a slight viewing condition change. During our experiments, we find all the three matching methods have similar distributions of their matching distances, even though they may fail in some cases.

Consequently, we evaluate their matching performance according to the geometrical shape of the detected regions. The matching results are classified into three levels: "GOOD," "OK," and "FAIL." Figure 6.20 gives an example for the three levels. If all of the content in the predefined region can be detected, we think this matching is "GOOD." For the "OK" level, the region is partially matched and influenced by its surroundings. If the methods cannot find the matching region, we think they "FAIL" the matching.

The performances of all three approaches within a predefined region are listed in Table 6.5. We tested six grouped emulated cases with slight viewing condition changes. These changes include planar translation (Emulated no. 1), planar rotation (Emulated no. 6), planar transform (Emulated no.

TABLE 6.5 Matching Performances of SIFT, SURF, and ORB Methods in Emulated *In Vitro* Testing Images

Group	SIFT	SURF	ORB
Emulated no. 1	OK	GOOD	FAIL
Emulated no. 2	GOOD	GOOD	OK
Emulated no. 3	GOOD	GOOD	FAIL
Emulated no. 4	GOOD	GOOD	OK
Emulated no. 5	OK	GOOD	FAIL
Emulated no. 6	GOOD	OK	GOOD

2), planar transform and background change (Emulated no. 5), zooming in (Emulated no. 3), and zooming out (Emulated no. 4). To create these changes, we either move the testing objects or change the endoscope pose. The matched features and regions of Emulated no. 1 and Emulated no. 2 are displayed in Figures 6.21 through 6.23. The regions of interest are highlighted using green contours. The well-matched feature points are connected by blue lines. According to the homography transform from these well-matched feature points, the same region can be detected in the target image.

For region matching in the *in vivo* surgical case, the three algorithms were validated under 10 groups of image pairs captured from 10 endoscopic surgical video clips. Taking into account the complexity of a real surgical scene, which may contain interference such as blood and smoke, we assume the image pairs will have just a slight viewing condition change. The matching performances of all the three methods are listed in Table 6.6. The target regions in these image pairs involve various viewing condition changes such as translation, rotation, planar transform, deformation, viewpoint change, zooming in/out, and occlusion. We classify these changes by observing the relevant positions of the target object in image pairs. Figures 6.24 through 6.26 display the matching results for the surgical video streams Real no. 2 and Real no. 3.

The following shows the experimental results of user-defined region matching using footage from both *in vitro* (Figure 6.27) and *in vivo* (Figure 6.28) endoscopic video streams.

The AR implementation was tested in a general environment and an emulated *in vitro* surgical environment. First, using surgical tools, the user selects a region in the surgical scene. Then a 3-D virtual object is overlaid on the selected region. When the view of the selected region is adjusted through movement of the endoscope, the region alignment algorithm can register the same region in different frames and render the virtual object on top of the matched region accordingly (Figure 6.29).

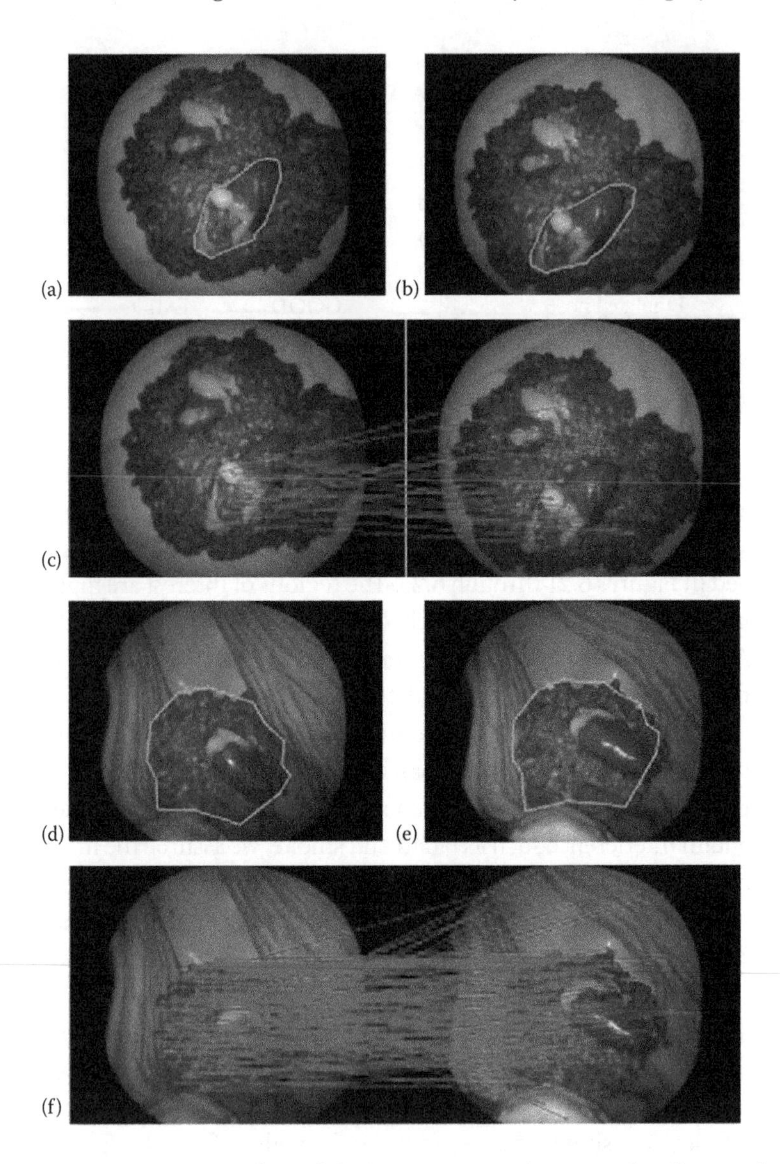

FIGURE 6.21 Two examples of SIFT region-matching results for emulated *in vitro* scenes: (a) and (d) are the source images with user-defined regions; (b) and (e) are the target images with detected regions.

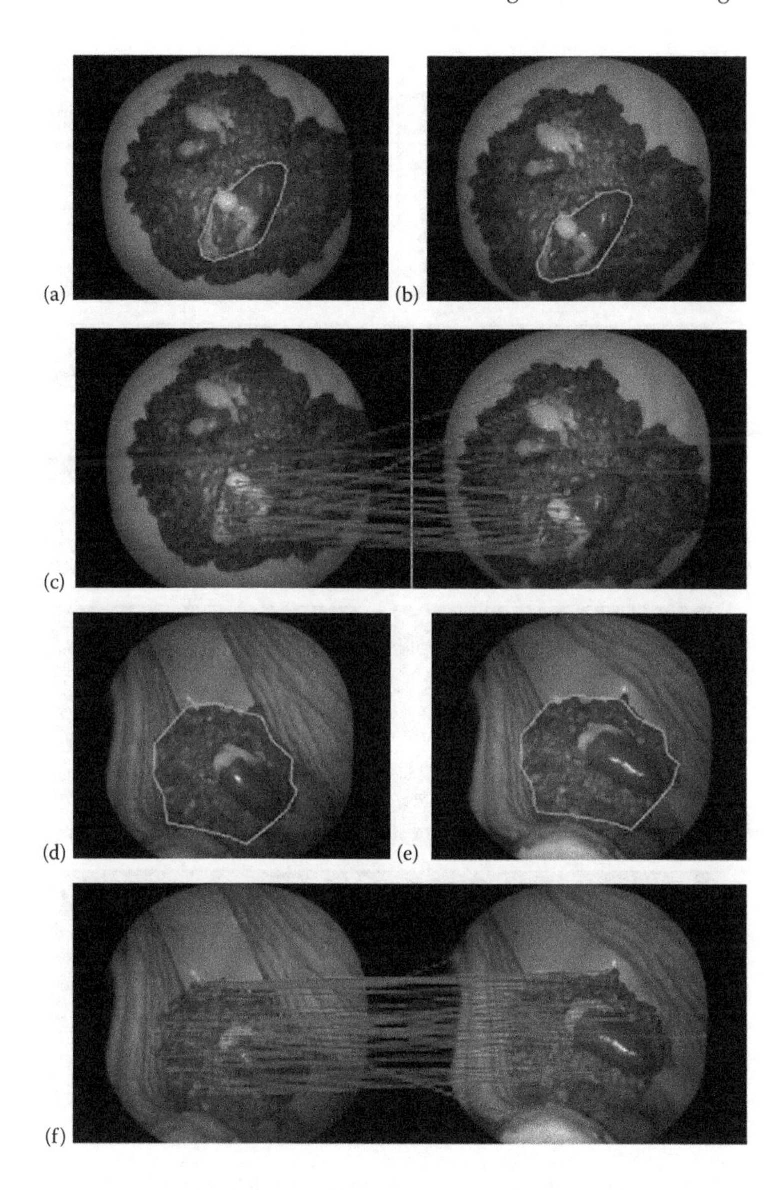

FIGURE 6.22 (a–c) and (d–f) are two examples of SURF region-matching results for emulated *in vitro* scenes.

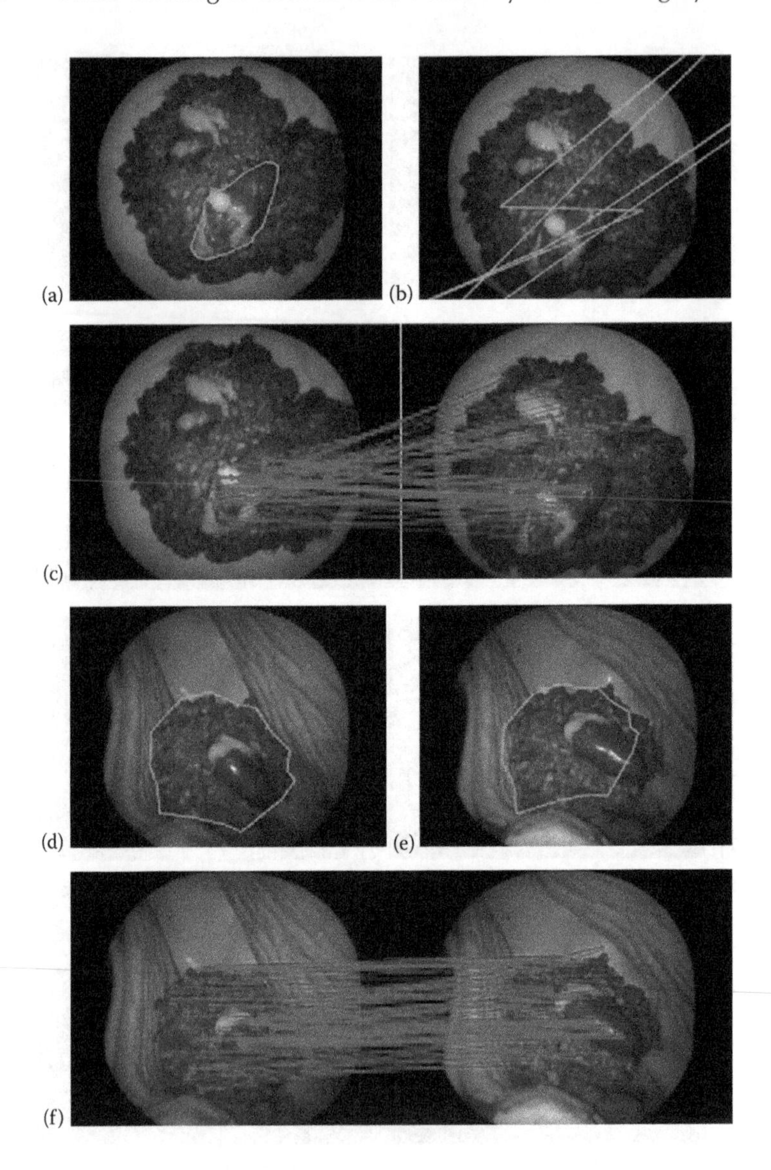

FIGURE 6.23 (a–c) and (d–f) are two examples of ORB region-matching results for emulated *in vitro* scenes.

TABLE 6.6 Matching Performances of SIFT, SURF, and ORB Methods Using Endoscopic Images of Surgical Scenes

Group	Region	Description	SIFT	SURF	ORB
Real no. 1	Polyp	Transform	GOOD	GOOD	GOOD
Real no. 2	Polyp	Transform	GOOD	GOOD	GOOD
Real no. 3	Vessel area	Zoom out	GOOD	OK	FAIL
Real no. 4	Bleeding tissue	Deformation and occlusion	GOOD	OK	FAIL
Real no. 5	Tissue	Translation	GOOD	OK	OK
Real no. 6	Tissue	Rotation	GOOD	GOOD	GOOD
Real no. 7	Tissue	Viewpoint change	GOOD	FAIL	FAIL
Real no. 8	Polyp	Rotation	GOOD	FAIL	OK
Real no. 9	Tissue	Occlusion	OK	FAIL	FAIL
Real no. 10	Bleeding tissue	Zoom in	GOOD	GOOD	OK

SUMMARY

In this chapter, three feature-based region alignment methods using SIFT, SURF, and ORB descriptors were presented. These methods were evaluated in a general environment, an emulated *in vitro* surgical environment, and a real surgical environment. For the general scenes, which contain sufficient feature structures, all the methods performed well on the user-defined region-matching tasks under different viewing conditions, with similar mean matching distances and standard deviations. In particular, the SIFT descriptor is invariant to most of the conditions, such as blurring, rotation, translation, exposure, planar transformation, and scaling (zooming in and out). However, it has the highest computational cost. In comparison, the SURF descriptor has a similar matching performance to the SIFT with a more practical computational speed. The ORB descriptor is superior to the SIFT and the SURF in computational cost, which satisfies the real-time requirement but has limitations in coping with scaling. The AR implementation was tested in a general environment and an emulated *in vitro* surgical environment. First, using surgical tools, the user selects a region in the surgical scene. Then a 3-D virtual object is overlaid on the selected region. When the view of the selected region is adjusted through movement of the endoscope, the region alignment algorithm can register the same region in different frames and render the virtual object on top of the matched region accordingly.

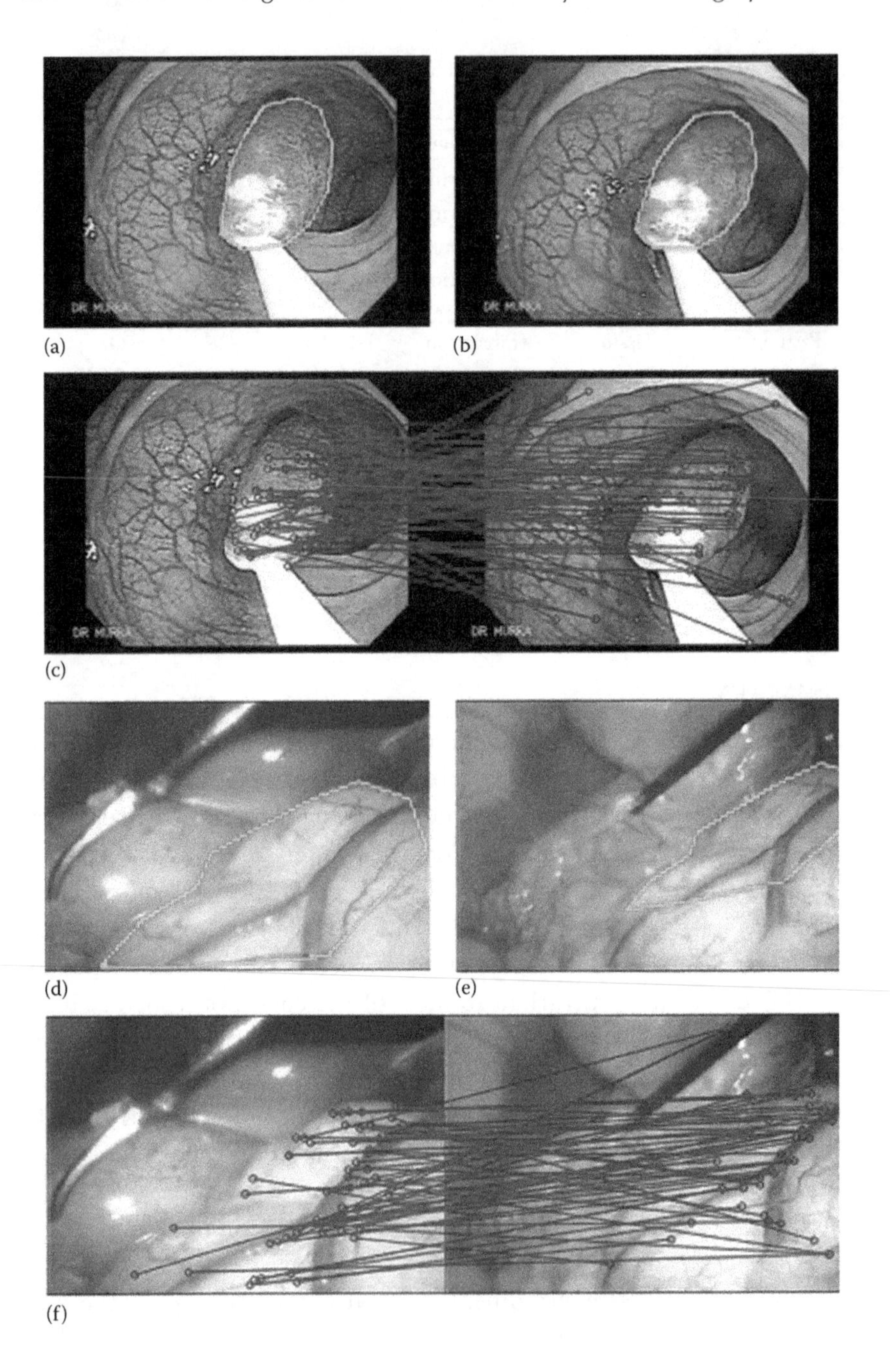

FIGURE 6.24 (a–c) and (d–f) are two examples of SIFT region-matching results for real surgical scenes: (a) and (d) are the source images with user-defined regions; (b) and (e) are the target images with detected regions.

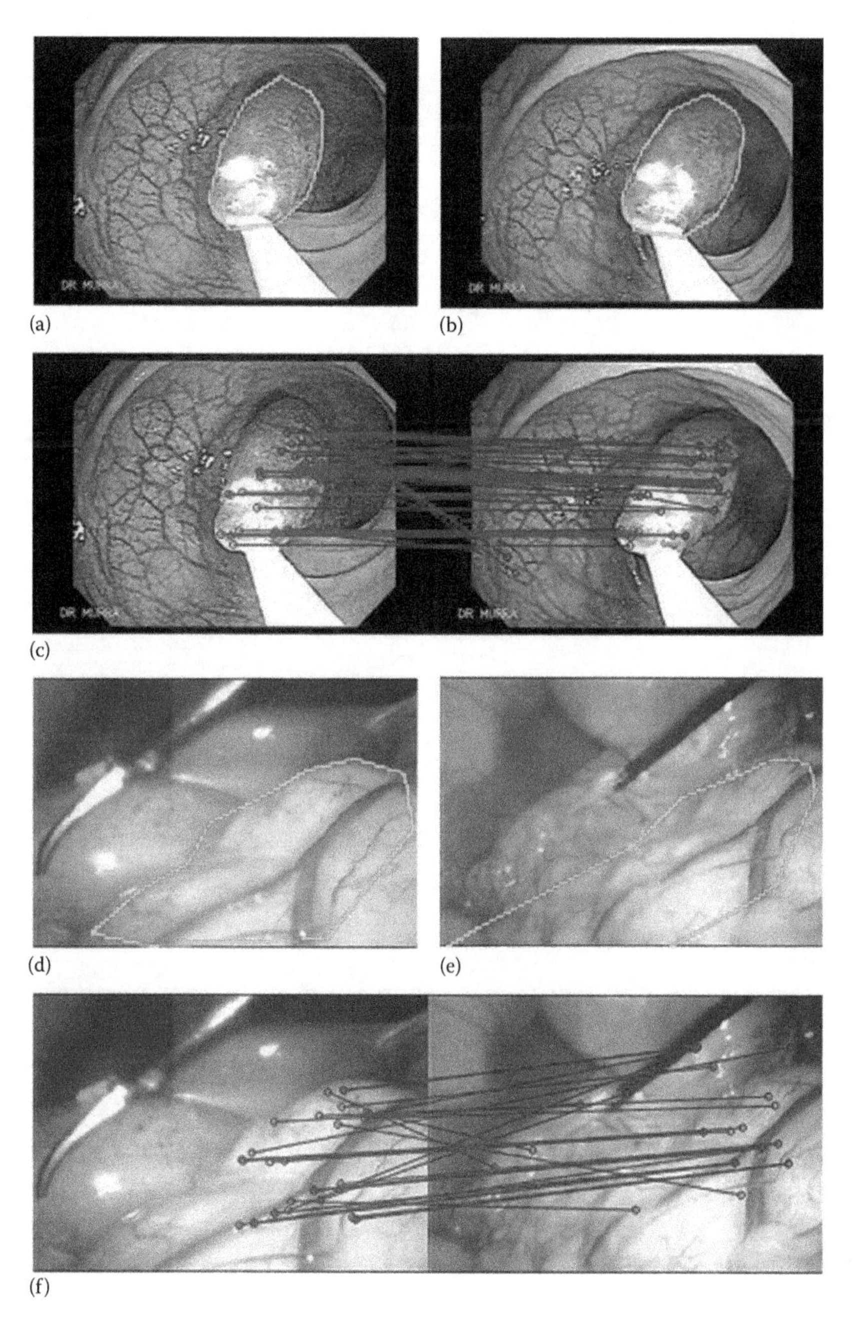

FIGURE 6.25 (a–c) and (d–f) are two examples of SURF region-matching results for endoscopic images of the surgical scenes.

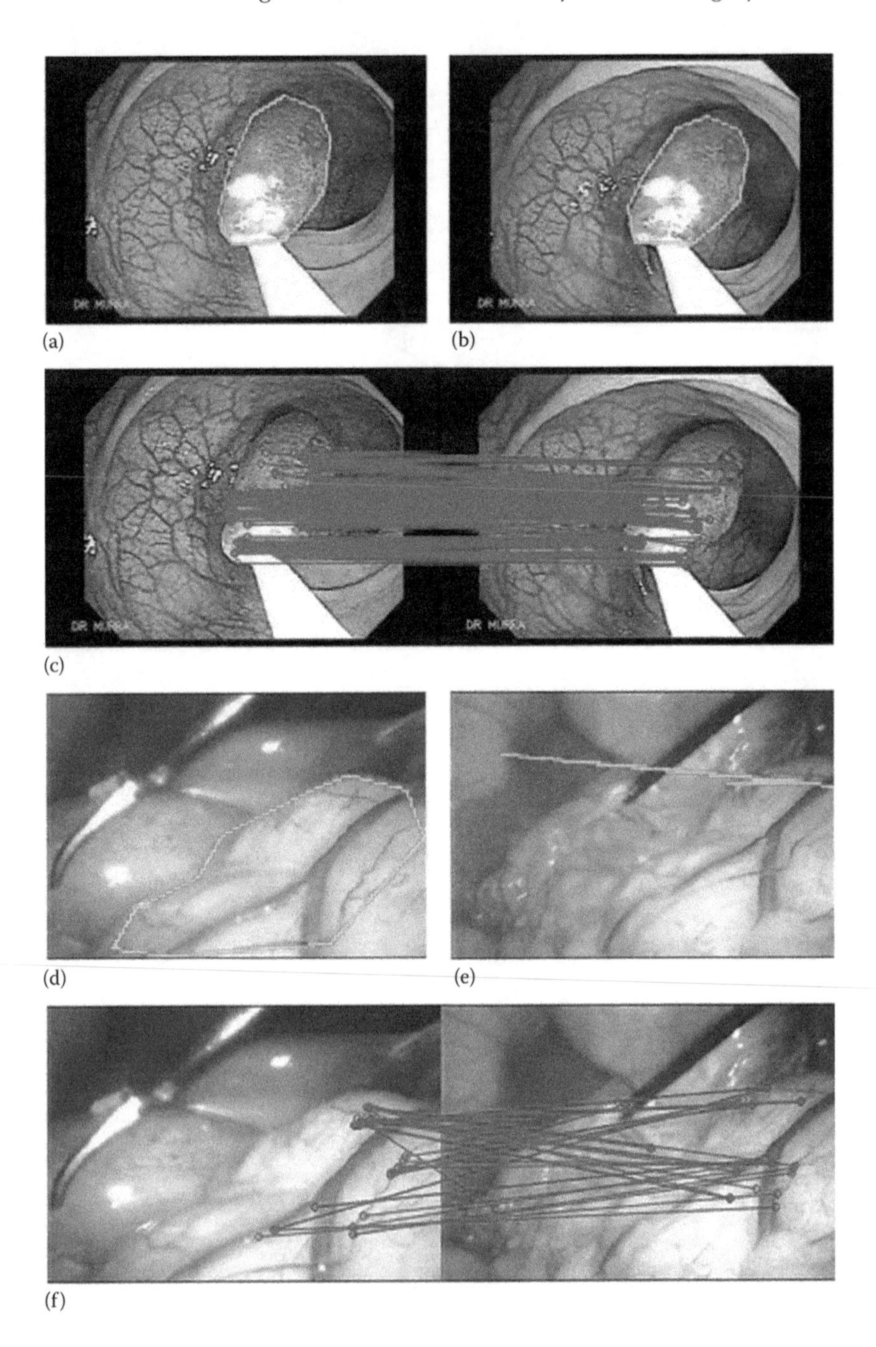

FIGURE 6.26 (a–c) and (d–f) are two examples of ORB region-matching results using the endoscopic images of the surgical scenes. (a) and (d) are the source images with the user defined regions. (b) and (e) are the target images with detected regions.

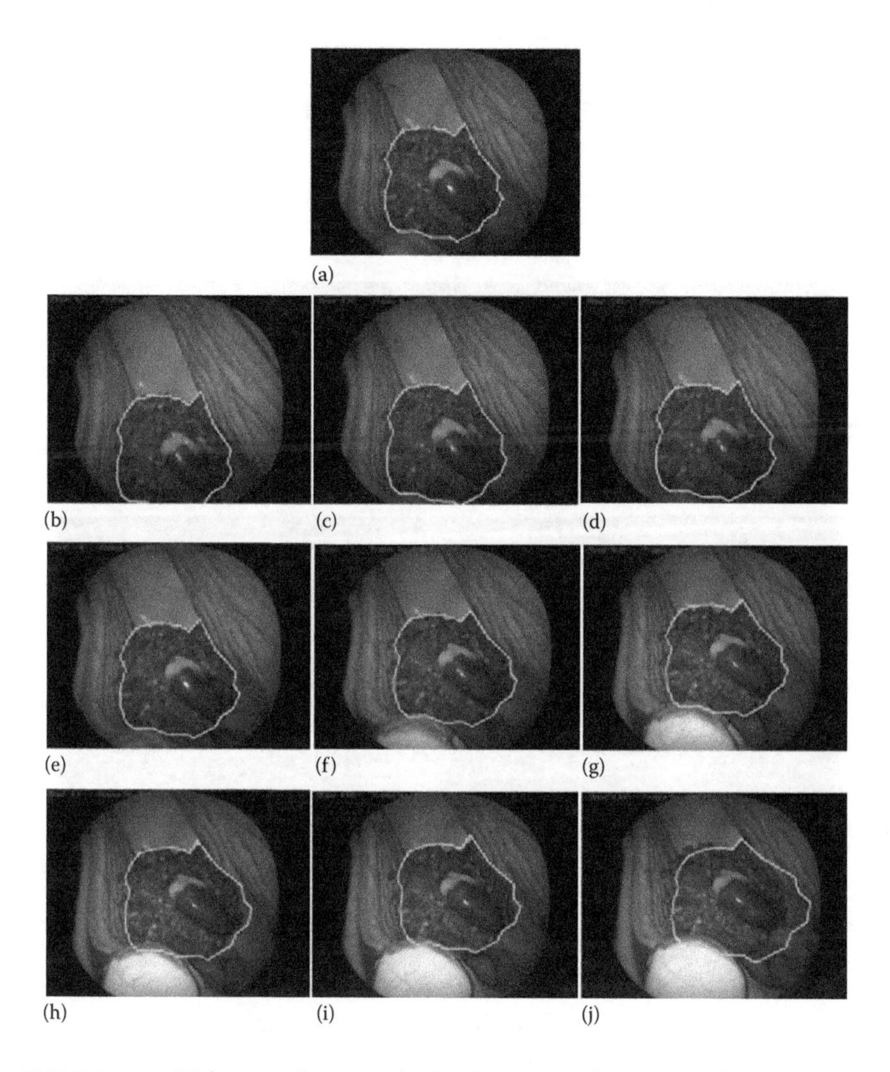

FIGURE 6.27 Video-matching results for the emulated *in vitro* endoscopic video stream using SURF matching. The user-defined region is highlighted by polygons. (a) User-defined region; (b) frame no. 134; (c) frame no. 139; (d) frame no. 145; (e) frame no. 148; (f) frame no. 154; (g) frame no. 165; (h) frame no. 170; (i) frame no. 177; (j) frame no. 183.

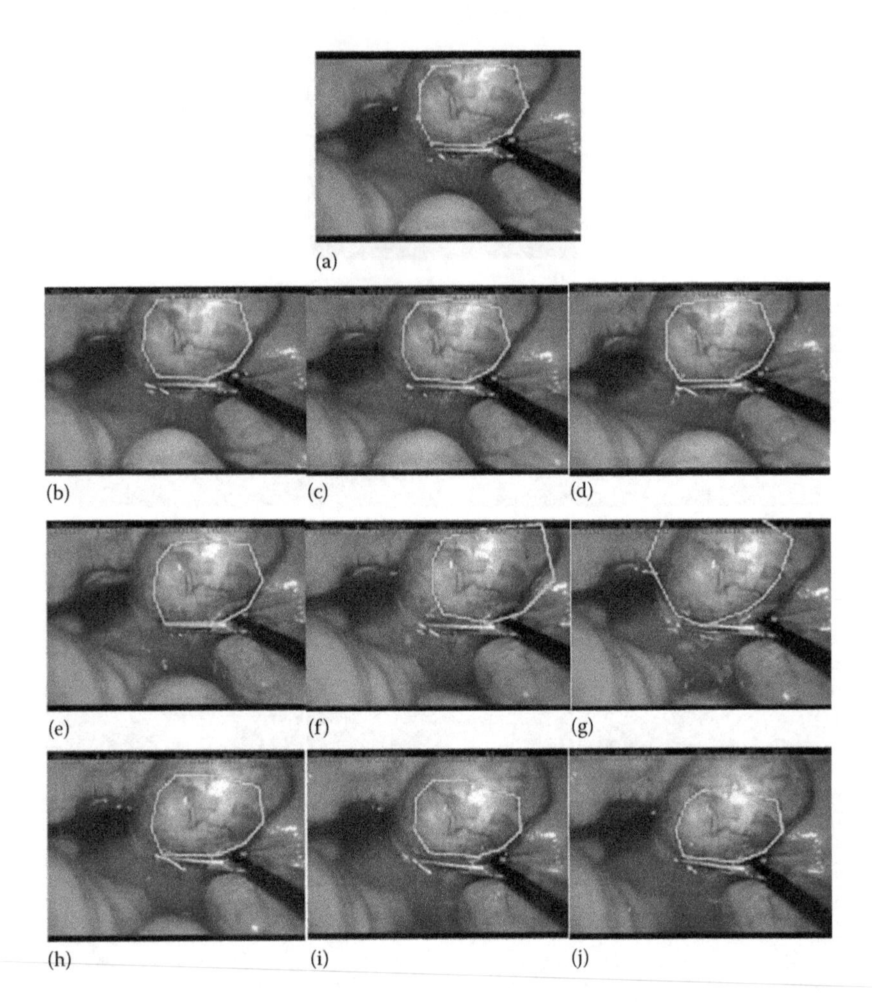

FIGURE 6.28 Video-matching results for the *in vivo* endoscopic video stream using SIFT matching. The user-defined region is highlighted by green polygon. (a) User-defined region; (b) frame no. 15; (c) frame no. 22; (d) frame no. 27; (e) frame no. 33; (f) frame no. 41; (g) frame no. 44; (h) frame no. 47; (i) frame no. 50; (j) frame no. 55.

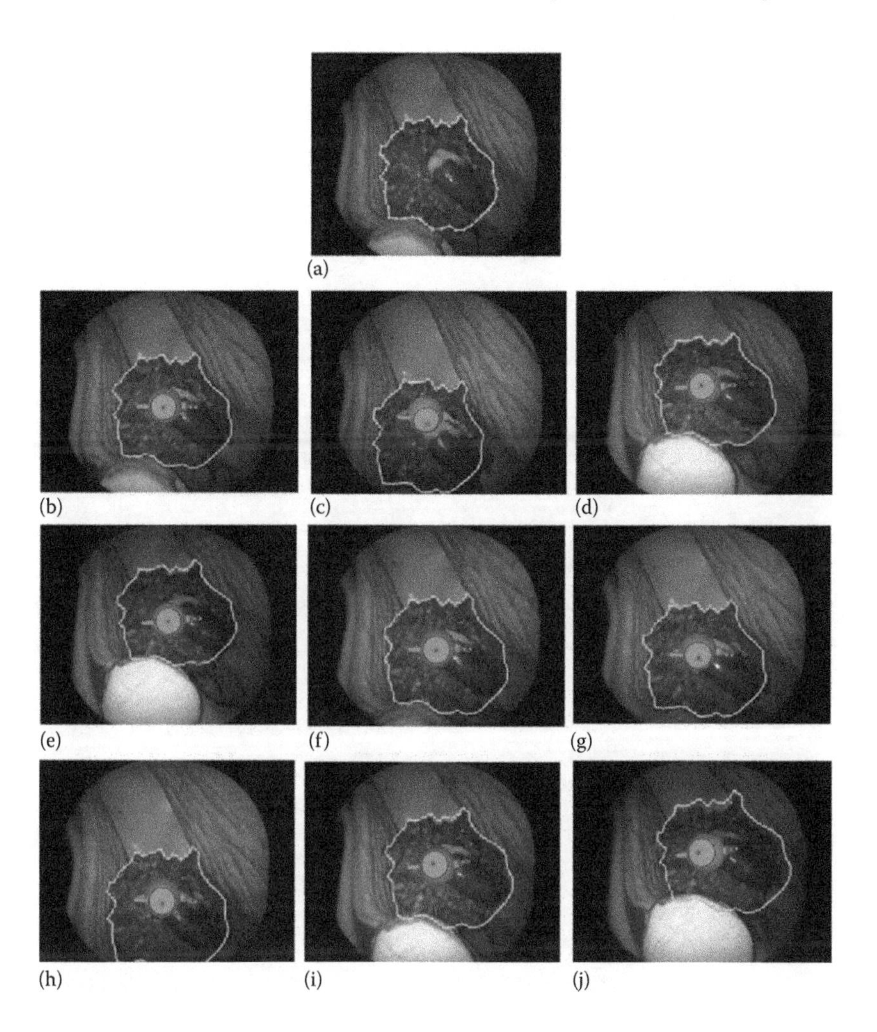

FIGURE 6.29 Example of AR demonstration for an emulated *in vitro* endoscopic video stream using the SURF region-matching approach. (a) User-defined region; (b) frame no. 49; (c) frame no. 109; (d) frame no. 184; (e) frame no. 227; (f) frame no. 306; (g) frame no. 358; (h) frame no. 380; (i) frame no. 423; (j) frame no. 451.

References

Ackermann, Ackermann finest surgical technology, http://www.ackermanninstrumente.de/index.html, last accessed February 2016.

Alahi, A., Ortiz, R., and Vandergheynst, P., FREAK: Fast retina keypoint, *Proceedings of IEEE Conference on Computer Vision and Pattern Recognition*, pp. 510–517, 2012.

Anzai, T. and Wang, J., A modified particle filter algorithm for wireless capsule endoscope location tracking, *Proceedings of the International Conference on Body Area Networks*, pp. 536–540, 2013.

Arulampalam, M.S., Maskell, S., Gordon, N. and Clapp, T., A tutorial on particle filters for on-line nonlinear/non-Gaussian Bayesian tracking, *IEEE Transaction on Signal Processing*, Vol. 50, No. 2, pp. 174–188, 2002.

Asari, K.V., Kumar, S., and Radhakrishnan, D., Technique of distortion correction in endoscopic images using a polynomial expansion, *Medical and Biological Engineering and Computing*, 37(1), 8–12, 1999.

Ascension, 3D guidance, http://www.ascension-tech.com/products, last accessed February 2016.

Bader, T., Wiedemann, A., Roberts, K., and Hanebeck, U.D., Model-based motion estimation of elastic surfaces for minimally invasive cardiac surgery, *Proceedings of IEEE International Conference on Robotic and Automation*, pp. 2261–2266, 2007.

Baek, S.J., Kim, J.S., Shin, J.W., and Kim, J., Robotic versus conventional laparoscopic surgery for rectal cancer: A cost analysis from a single institute in Korea, *Journal of World Surgery*, 36(11), 2722–2729, 2012.

Bay, H., Tuytelaars, T., and Van Gool, L., SURF: Speeded up robust features, In *Computer Vision: ECCV*, pp. 404–417, 2006.

BBC, Robotic surgery linked to 144 deaths in the US, http://www.bbc.com/news/technology-33609495, last accessed February 2016.

Bishop, C., *Neural Network for Pattern Recognition*, New York: Oxford University Press, 2005.

Bishop, C., *Pattern Recognition and Machine Learning*, New York, Springer, 2006.

Borkar, A., Hayes, M., and Smith, M.T., Robust lane detection and tracking with RANSAC and Kalman filter, *IEEE International Conference on Image Processing*, pp. 3261–3264, 2009.

Bouarfa, L., Akman, O., Schneider, A., Jonker, P., and Dankelman, J., In-vivo real-time tracking of surgical instruments in endoscopic video, *Minimally Invasive Therapy and Allied Technology*, 21(3), 129–134, 2012.

Bradski, G.R. and Davis, J.W., Motion segmentation and pose representation with motion history gradients, *Machine Vision and Applications*, 13(3), 174–184, 2002.

Breitenstein, M.D., Reichlin, F., Leibe, B., Van Gool, E.K., and Leuven, K.U., Robust tracking-by-detection using a detector confidence particle filter, *Proceedings of IEEE International Conference on Computer Vision*, pp. 1515–1522, 2009.

Brown, M. and Lowe, D., Invariant features from interest point groups, *Proceedings of British Machine Vision Conference*, pp. 656–665, 2002.

Calonder, M., Lepetit, V., Strecha, C., and Fua, P., BRIEF: Binary robust independent elementary features, In *Computer Vision: ECCV*, pp. 778–792, 2010.

Canny, J., A computational approach to edge detection, *IEEE Transactions on Pattern Analysis and Machine Intelligence*, 8(6), 679–698, 1986.

Cano, A.M., Gaya, F., Lamata, P., Sanchez-Gonzalez, P., and Gomez, E.J., Laparoscopic tool tracking method for augmented reality surgical applications, In *Biomedical Simulation*, pp. 191–196, 2008.

Cano, A.M., Lamata, P., Gay, F., and Gmez, E., New method for video-based tracking of laparoscopic tools, In *Biomedical Simulation*, pp. 142–149, 2006.

Chen, C., Stitt, S., and Zheng, Y.F., Robotic eye-in-hand calibration by calibrating optical axis and target pattern, *Journal of Intelligent and Robotic System*, 12, 155–173, 1995.

Climent, J. and Hexsel, R., Particle filtering in the Hough space for instrument tracking, *The International Journal of Computers in Biology and Medicine*, 24(5), 614–623, 2012.

ClinicalTrials.gov (US National Institute of Health), 3D vs 2D laparoscopy in cholecystectomy, https://clinicaltrials.gov/ct2/show/NCT02357589, last accessed February 2016.

Comanicui, D., Ramesh, V., and Meer, P., Kernel-based object tracking, *IEEE Transactions on Pattern Analysis and Machine Intelligence*, 25(5), 564–577, 2003.

Daga, B., Bhute, A., and Ghato, A., Implementation of parallel image processing using NVIDIA GPU framework: In *Advanced in Computing, Communication and Control*, pp. 457–464, 2011.

Dai, X. and Payandeh, S., Geometry-based object association and consistent labeling in multi-camera surveillance, *IEEE Journal of Emerging and Selected Topics in Circuits and Systems*, 3(2), 175–184, 2013.

Davis, J.W., Hierarchical motion history images for recognizing human motion, *IEEE Workshop on Detection and Recognition of Events in Video*, pp. 39–46, 2001.

Dellaert, F. and Thorpe, C., Robust car tracking using Kalman filtering and Bayesian templates, *Proceedings of Conference on Intelligent Transportation Systems*, SPIE, Vol. 3207, 1997.

Doignon, C., Greabling, P., and Mathelin, M., Real-time segmentation of surgical instruments inside the abdominal cavity using a join hue saturation color feature, *Real-Time Imaging*, 11, 429–442, 2005.

FANN, Fast artificial neural network library, http://leenissen.dk/fann/wp, last accessed February 2016.

Faraz, A. and Payandeh, S., Adjustable surgical stand, US Patent 5,824,007, 1998.

Faraz, A. and Payandeh, S., *Engineering Approaches to Mechanical and Robotic Design for Minimally Invasive Surgery*, Boston, MA, Kluwer Academic Publishers, 2000.

Fischler, M. and Bolles, R., Random sample consensus: A paradigm for model fitting with applications to image analysis and automated cartography, *Communication of ACM*, 24(6), 381–395, 1981.

FLS, FLS trainer box, Limbs & Things, http://www.fls-products.com/home, last accessed February 2016.

Fu, X. and Han, Y., Centroid weighted Kalman filter for visual object tracking, *Measurement*, 45(4), 650–655, 2012.

Funda, J., LaRose, D.A., and Taylor, R., Robotic system for positioning a surgical instrument relative to a patient's body, US Patent 5,527,999, 1996.

Gaschler, A., Burschka, D., and Hager, G., Epipolar-based stereo tracking without explicit 3d reconstruction, *Proceedings of International Conference on Pattern Recognition*, pp. 1755–1758, 2010.

Giannarou, S., Visentini-Scarzanella, M., and Yang, G.Z., Probabilistic tracking of affine-invariant anisotropic regions, *IEEE Transactions on Pattern Analysis and Machine Intelligence*, 35(1), 130–143, 2013.

Gonzalez, C. and Wood, R., *Digital Image Processing*, Englewood Cliffs, NJ, Prentice Hall, 2002.

Grimson, W.E., Stauffer, C., and Lee, L., Using adaptive tracking to classify and monitor activities is a site, *Proceedings of IEEE Conference on Computer Vision and Pattern Recognition*, pp. 22–29, 1998.

Guha, S., *Computer Graphics through OpenGL: From Theory to Experiments*, Boca Raton, FL, CRC Press, 2015.

Hartley, R. and Zisserman, A., *Multiple View Geometry in Computer Vision*, Cambridge, Cambridge University Press, 2006.

Hatada, Y., Iwane, S., Tohno, H., Baba, T., Munakata, A., and Yoshida, Y., A new method for measurement of the gastric and colonic lesions with an electronic endoscope and image processor, *Gastrointestinal Endoscopy*, 37, 275–281, 1991.

Heinly, J., Dunn, E., and Frahm, J., Comparative evaluation of binary features, In *Computer Vision: ECCV*, pp. 759–773, 2012.

Hough, P., Method and means for recognizing complex patterns, US Patent 3,069,654, 1962.

Hsu, J., Toward integration of a surgical robotic system with automatic tracking, tool, gesture and motion recognition, MASc. thesis, Burnaby, BC, Simon Fraser University, 2007.

Hsu, J. and Payandeh, S., Toward toll gesture and motion recognition on a novel minimally invasive surgery robotics system, *Proceedings of IEEE International Conference on Robotics and Automation*, pp. 631–637, 2006.

Huang, C.C., Hung, N.M., and Kumar, A. Hybrid method for 3D instrument reconstruction and tracking in laparoscopic surgery, *International Conference on Control, Automation and Information Science*, pp. 36–41, 2013.

Intuitive Surgical, The da Vinci System, http://www.intuitivesurgical.com/company, last accessed February 2016.

JHN, Use of minimally invasive surgery could lower health care costs by hundreds of millions a year, http://www.hopkinsmedicine.org/news/media/releases, last accessed February 2016.

Kaewtrakulpong, P. and Bowden, R., An improved adaptive background mixture model for real-time tracking with shadow detection, In *Video-Based Surveillance Systems*, pp. 135–144, 2002.

Kang, B., Tripathi, S., and Nguyen, T., Real-time sign language finger spelling recognition using conventional neural networks from depth map, *Proceedings of IAPR Conference on Pattern Recognition*, 2015.

Kass, M., Witkin, A., and Terzopoulos, D., Snakes: Active contour models, *International Journal of Computer Vision*, 1(4), 321–331, 1988.

Khong, W., Kow, W., Wong, F., Saad, I., and Teo, K., Enhancement of particle filter approach for vehicle tracking via adaptive resampling algorithm, *Proceedings of IEEE International Conference on Computational Intelligence, Communication Systems and Networks*, pp. 259–263, 2011.

Krupa, A., Member, A., Gangloff, J., Doignon, C., De Mathelin, M., Morel, G., Leroy, J., and Soler, L., Autonomous 3-D positioning of surgical instruments in robotized laparoscopic surgery using visual servoing, *IEEE Transactions on Robotics and Automation*, 19(5), 842–853, 2003.

LapMentor, Lap Mentor surgical simulator, http://simbionix.com/simulators/lap-mentor, last accessed February 2016.

LapTrainer, Laparoscopic trainer Abc-lap, http://www.lap-trainer.com/?pg=main, last accessed February 2016.

LeDuc, M., Payandeh, S. and Dill, J., Toward modeling of a suturing task, *Proceedings of Graphics Interface*, pp. 273–279, 2003.

Lee, J. and Payandeh, S., *Haptic Teleoperation Systems: Signal Processing Perspective*, Cham, Switzerland, Springer, 2015.

Leutenegger, S., Chli, M., and Siegwart, R.Y., BRISK: Binary robust invariant scalable keypoints, *Proceedings of IEEE International Conference on Computer Vision: ICCV*, pp. 2548–2555, 2011.

Li, B. and Meng, Q.H., Computer-aided detection of bleeding regions for capsule endoscopy images, *IEEE Transactions on Biomedical Engineering*, pp. 681–684, 2009.

Liu, W. and Vinter, B., An efficient GPU general sparse matrix–matrix multiplication for irregular data, *Proceedings of IEEE International Conference on Parallel and Distributed Processing*, pp. 370–381, 2014.

Loukas, C., An integrated approach to endoscopic instrument tracking for augmented reality applications in surgical simulation training, *The International Journal of Medical Robotics and Computer Assisted Surgery*, 9(4), 34–51, 2013.

Lowe, D.G., Distinctive image features from scale-invariant keypoints, *International Journal of Computer Vision*, 60(2), 91–110, 2004.

Lu, Y., Cooperative hybrid tracking for event monitoring systems, MASc. thesis, Burnaby, BC, Simon Fraser University, 2008.

Lu, Y. and Payandeh, S., Cooperative hybrid multi-camera tracking for people surveillance, *IEEE Canadian Journal of Electrical and Computer Engineering*, 33(3), 145–152, 2008.

Ma, Z. and Ujiki, M.B., Surgical resident evaluation of portable laparoscopic box trainers incorporated into a simulation-based minimally invasive surgery, *Surgical Innovation*, 22(1), 83–87, 2015.

Marchand, E., Spindler, F., and Chaumette, F., ViSP for visual servoing: A generic software platform with a wide class of robot control skills, *IEEE Robotics and Automation Magazine*, 12(4), 40–52, 2005.

Margulies, C., Krevsky, B., and Catalano, M.F., How accurate are endoscopic estimates of size? *Gastrointestinal Endoscopy*, 40, 174–177, 1994.

McKenna, S.J., Charif, H.N., and Frank, T., Toward video understanding of laparoscopic surgery, *Proceedings of Image and Vision Computing*, 2005.

Mikolajczyk, K., Tuytelaars, T., Schmid, C., Zisserman, A., Matas, J., Schaffalitzky, F., Kadir, T., and Van Gool, L., A comparison of affine region detectors, *International Journal of Computer Vision*, 65(1), 43–72, 2005.

Mills, S., Pridmore, T.P., and Hills, M., Tracking in a Hough space with the extended Kalman filter, *Proceedings of British Machine Vision Conference*, pp. 18.1–18.10, 2003.

Muja, M. and Lowe, D.G., Fast approximate nearest neighbors with automatic algorithm configuration, *Proceedings of the International Conference on Computer Vision Theory and Applications*, pp. 331–340, 2009.

Nadler, M. and Smith, E.O., *Pattern Recognition Engineering*, New York, Wiley, 1993.

Nummiaro, K., Koller-Meier, E., and Van Gool, L., An adaptive color-based particle filter, *Image and Vision Computing*, 21(1), 99–110, 2003.

OpenNN, Open Neural Networks Library, http://opennn.cimne.com, last accessed February 2016.

Ortmaier, T., Groger, M., Boehm, D.H., Falk, V., and Hirzinger, G., Motion estimation in beating heart surgery, *IEEE Transactions on Biomedical Engineering*, 52(10), 1729–1740, 2005.

Parada, R. and Payandeh, S., On study of design and implementation of virtual fixtures, *Virtual Reality*, 14(2), 117–129, 2009.

Payandeh, S., Design of a multi-modal dexterity training interface for medical and biological science, In *Holistic Perspectives in Gamification for Clinical Practice*, pp. 536–564, 2015.

Payandeh, S., Hsu, J., and Doris, P., Toward the design of a novel surgeon computer interface using image processing of surgical tools in minimally invasive surgery, *The International Journal of Medical Engineering and Informatics*, 4(1), 1–24, 2012.

Payandeh, S. and Li, T., Toward new design of haptic devices for minimally invasive surgery, *Proceedings of Computer Assisted Radiology and Surgery*, pp. 775–781, 2003.

Payandeh, S. and Shi, H., Interactive multi-modal suturing, *Virtual Reality*, 14(4), 241–253, 2010.

Pratt, P., Stoyanov, D., Visentini-Scarzanella, M., and Yang, G.Z., Dynamic guidance for robotic surgery using image-constrained biomechanical models, In *Medical Image Computing and Computer-Assisted Intervention*, pp. 77–85, 2010.

Rehg, J.M. and Kanada, T., Model-based tracking of self-occluding articulated objects, *Proceedings of International Conference on Computer Vision*, pp. 612–617, 1995.

Reiter, A., Allen, P.K., and Zhao, T., Feature classification for tracking articulated surgical tools, In *Medical Image Computing and Computer-Assisted Intervention*, pp. 592–600, 2012.

Rigatos, G.G., Nonlinear Kalman filters and practical filters for integrated navigation of unmanned aerial vehicles, *Robotics and Autonomous Systems*, 60(7), 978–995, 2012.

Ristic, B., Arulampalam, S., and Gordon, N., *Beyond the Kalman Filter: Particle Filters for Tracking Applications*, Boston, MA, Artech House Publishing, 2004.

Rosin, P., Measuring corner properties, *Computer Vision and Image Understanding*, 73(2), 291–307, 1999.

Ross, D., Lim, J., Lin, R., and Yang, M., Incremental learning for robust visual tracking, *International Journal of Computer Vision*, 77(1), 125–141, 2008.

Rosten, E. and Drummond, T., Machine learning for high-speed corner detection, In *Computer Vision: ECCV*, pp. 430–443, 2006.

Rublee, E., Garage, W., and Park, M., ORB: An efficient alternative to SIFT or SURF, *Proceedings of IEEE International Conference on Computer Vision*, pp. 2564–2571, 2011.

Ryu, J., Choi, J., and Kim, H.C., Endoscopic vision-based tracking of multiple surgical instruments during robot-assisted surgery, *Artificial Organs*, 37(1), 107–112, 2013.

Sages, Society of American Gastrointestinal and Endoscopic Surgeons, http://www.sages.org, last accessed February 2016.

Sahoo, P., Soltani, S., Wong, A., and Chen, Y., A survey of thresholding techniques, *Computer Vision, Graphics, and Image Processing*, 41(2), 233–260, 1988.

Sa-Ing, V., Thongvigitmanee, S.S., Wilasrusmee, C., and Suthakorn, J., Object tracking for laparoscopic surgery using the adaptive mean-shift Kalman algorithm, *International Journal of Machine Learning and Computing*, 1(5), 441–447, 2011.

Salajegheh, M., Imaging of surgical tools as a new paradigm for surgeon computer-interface in minimally invasive surgery, MASc. thesis, Burnaby, BC, Simon Fraser University, 2008.

Salembier, P. and Pardas, M., Hierarchy morphological segmentation for image sequence coding, *IEEE Transactions on Image Processing*, 2(5), 639–651, 1994.

Sarlos, D., Kots, L., Stevanovic, N., Von Felten, S., and Schar, G., Robotics compared with conventional laparoscopic hysterectomy: A randomized controlled trial, *Journal of Obstetrics and Gynecology*, 120(3), 640–611, 2012.

Schafer, R.W. and Lawrence, R.R., A digital signal processing approach to interpolation, *Proceedings of IEEE*, 61, 692–702, 1973.

Seal, Seal open and endoscopic surgery trainer, http://seal.se, last accessed February 2016.

Shi, F. and Payandeh, S., GPU in haptic rendering of deformable objects, In *Haptics: Perception, Devices and Scenarios*, pp. 163–168, 2008.

Shi, F. and Payandeh, S., Interactive multi-modal suturing, *Virtual Reality*, 14(4), 241–253, 2010.

Shimada, M., Iwasaki, S., and Asakura, T., Finger spelling recognition using neural network with pattern recognition, *Proceedings of IEEE SICE Conference*, pp. 2458–2463, 2003.

Shin, S., Kim, Y., Kwak, H., Lee, D., and Park, S., 3D tracking of surgical instruments using a single camera for laparoscopic surgery simulation, *Studies in Health Technology and Informatics*, 163, 581–587, 2010.

Singla, A., Li, Y., Ng, S.C., Csikesz, N.G., Tseng, J.F., and Shah, S.A., Is the growth in laparoscopic surgery reproducible with more complex procedures? *Surgery*, 146(2), 367–374, 2009.

Smith, W.E., Vakil, N., and Maislin, S.A., Correction of distortion in endoscope images, *IEEE Transactions on Medical Imaging*, 11(1), 117–122, 1992.

Sousa, A., Areia, M., and Coimbra, M., Identifying cancer regions in vital-stained magnification endoscopy images using adapted color histogram, *Proceedings of IEEE International Conference on Image Processing*, pp. 681–684, 2009.

Spaner, S. and Warnock, G., A brief history of endoscopy, laparoscopy, and laparoscopic surgery, *Journal of Laparoendoscopic and Advanced Surgical Techniques*, 7(6), 369–373, 2009.

Speidel, S., Delles, M., Gutt, C., and Dillmann, R., Tracking of instruments in minimally invasive surgery for surgical skill analysis, In *Medical Imaging and Augmented Reality*, pp. 148–155, 2006.

Stergiou, C. and Siganos, D., Neural networks, http://www.doc.ic.ac.uk/~nd/surprise_96/journal/vol4/cs11/report.html, last accessed February 2016.

Storz, Karl Storz endoscope, https://www.karlstorz.com/ca/en/index.htm, last accessed February 2016.

Stoyanov, D., Darzi, A., and Yang, G.Z., Dense 3D depth recovery for soft tissue deformation during robotically assisted laparoscopic surgery, In *Medical Image Computing and Computer-Assisted Intervention*, pp. 41–48, 2004.

Stoyanov, D. and Yang, G.Z., Soft tissue deformation tracking for robotic assisted minimally invasive surgery, *Proceedings of IEEE International Conference on Engineering in Medicine and Biology*, pp. 254–257, 2009.

Strecha, C., Von Hansen, W., Van Gool, L., and Fua, P., On benchmarking camera calibration and multi-view stereo for high resolution imagery, *Proceedings of IEEE Conference on Vision and Pattern Recognition*, pp. 1–8, 2008.

Sun, X., Image guided interaction in minimally invasive surgery, MASc. thesis, Burnaby, BC, Simon Fraser University, 2012.

Sun, X. and Payandeh, S., Toward design and development of surgeon computer interface, *Proceedings of the IASTED International Conference Robotics and Applications*, pp. 115–121, 2011a.

Sun, X. and Payandeh, S., Toward development of 3D surgical mouse paradigm, *Proceedings of IEEE/RSJ International Conference on Intelligent Robotic System*, pp. 2096–2101, 2011b.

Tai, J. and Song, K., Background segmentation and its application to traffic monitoring using modified histogram, *IEEE International Conference on Networking, Sensing and Control*, Vol. 1, pp. 13–18, 2004.

Tanimoto, S.L., *An Interdisciplinary Introduction to Image Processing: Pixel, Numbers and Programs*, Cambridge, MA, MIT Press, 2012.

Tehrani Niknejad, H., Takeuchi, A., Mita, S., and McAllester, D., On-road multivehicle tracking using deformable object and particle filter with improved likelihood estimation, *IEEE Transactions on Intelligent Transportation System*, 13(2), 748–758, 2012.

Tonet, O., Thoranaghatte, R., Megali, G., and Dario, P., Tracking endoscopic instruments without a localizer, *Computer Aided Surgery*, 12(1), 35–42, 2007.

Tsai, R.Y., A versatile camera calibration technique for high-accuracy 3D machine vision metrology using off-the-shelf TV cameras and lenses, *IEEE Journal of Robotics and Automation*, RA-3(4), 323–344, 1987.

Viola, O. and Jones, M., Rapid object detection using a boosted cascade of simple feature, *Proceedings of IEEE Conference on Computer Vision and Pattern Recognition*, pp. 511–518, 2001.

Visionsense, VSiii System, http://www.visionsense.com/vsiii-system, last accessed February 2016.

Voisin, V., Avila, M., Emile, B., and Begot, S., Road marking detection and tracking using Hough transform and Kalman filter, In *Advanced Concepts for Intelligent Vision Systems*, pp. 76–83, 2005.

Wei, G. and Arbter, K., Automatic tracking of laparoscopic instruments by color coding, *First Joint Conference Computer Vision, Virtual Reality and Robotics in Medicine and Medical Robotics and Computer-Assisted Surgery*, pp. 19–22, 1997.

Wolf, P.R., *Elements of Photogrammetry*, New York, McGraw-Hill, 1983.

Wright, J.D., Ananth, C.V., Lewin, S.N., Burke, W.M., Lu, Y.S., Neugun, A.I., Herzon, T.J., and Hershman, D.L., Robotically assisted vs laparoscopic hysterectomy among women with benign gynecologic disease, *The Journal of American Medical Association*, 309(7), 689–698, 2013.

Xuan, J., Adali, T., and Wang, Y., Automatic detection of foreign objects in computed radiology, *IEEE International Conference on Engineering in Medicine and Biology*, pp. 719–721, 1998.

Yang, B., Pan, X., Men, A., and Chen, X., A robust particle filter for people tracking, *Proceedings of IEEE International Conference on Future Networks*, pp. 20–23, 2010.

Yip, M.C., Lowe, D.G., Salcudean, S.E., Rohling, R.N., and Nguan, C.Y., Real-time methods for long-term tissue feature tracking in endoscopic scenes, In *Information Processing in Computer-Assisted Interventions*, pp. 33–43, 2012.

Zarchan, P. and Musoff, H., *Fundamentals of Kalman Filtering: A Practical Approach*, Vol. 232, Progress in Astronautics and Aeronautics, Reston, VA, American Institute of Aeronautics and Astronautics, 2009.

Zhang, X., Application of image tracking and 3D image reconstruction for laparoscopic surgery, MASc. thesis, Burnaby, BC, Simon Fraser University, 2002.

Zhang, X. and Payandeh, S., Application of visual tracking for robot-assisted laparoscopic surgery, *Journal of Robotic Systems*, 19(7), 315–328, 2002.

Zhou, J., Visual tracking and region alignment in surgical and medical education, MASc. thesis, Burnaby, BC, Simon Fraser University, 2014.

Zhou, J. and Payandeh, S., Visual tracking of laparoscopic instruments, *Journal of Automation and Control Engineering*, 2(3), 234–241 2014.

Zhou, J. and Payandeh, S., An experimental study of visual tracking in surgical applications, *Proceedings of the International Conference on Computer Vision Theory and Applications*, pp. 608–613, 2015a.

Zhou, J. and Payandeh, S., On user-defined region matching for augmented reality, *Proceedings of IEEE Canadian Conference on Electrical and Computer Engineering*, pp. 1414–1419, 2015b.

Appendix I: Lens Distortion Model

For field data containing random errors, a process of quantitatively estimating the trend of the outcomes, also known as *regression* or *curve fitting*, is often used.

The curve fitting process fits equations for approximating curves to the raw field data. Nevertheless, for a given set of data, the fitting curves of a given type are generally not unique. Thus, a curve with a minimal deviation from all data points is desired. *Least squares* is a procedure to obtain the best-fitting curve.

As described in Chapter 2, the $M+1$ deviation equations can be represent in matrix form:

$$AK = Y \tag{I.1}$$

where:

$$A = \left[r_i^{2j+1}\right]_{(M+1)\times(M+1)}, \text{for } i = 0,\ldots M,\ j = 0,\ldots, M$$

$$K = \left[k_0, k_1, \ldots, k_M\right]^T$$

$$Y = \left[y_0, y_1, \ldots, y_M\right]^T$$

Equation I.1 can be written as

$$A^T AK = A^T Y \tag{I.2}$$

Multiply both sides of Equation I.2 by $(A^T A)^{-1}$ and, simplifying, we can obtain

$$K = (A^T A)^{-1} A^T Y \quad (I.3)$$

In the following example, a practical application of the image distortion correction method is presented (see Table AI.1). The following form is used to define radial lens distortions:

$$\Delta r = k_1 r + k_2 r^3 \quad (I.4)$$

In Equation I.4, Δr is the radial-lens distortion at a radial distance r from the principal point. The k's are coefficients that define the shape of the radial lens distortion and a third-order polynomial.

From the experiment data, five equations can be obtained in terms of k values that can be computed by the least squares method.

$$0 = (28)k_1 + (28)^3 k_2$$

$$1 = (56)k_1 + (56)^3 k_2$$

$$2 = (84)k_1 + (84)^3 k_2$$

$$4 = (112)k_1 + (112)^3 k_2$$

$$6 = (140)k_1 + (140)^3 k_2$$

TABLE AI.1 Lens Distortion Correction Data

Radial Distance *r* (Pixel)	**Radial Lens Distortion (Pixel)**
28	0
56	1
84	2
112	4
140	6

Using the least squares method for solution of Equation I.3, the following values were obtained for the two coefficients:

$$k_1 = 0.013084138 \qquad k_2 = 0.000001575$$

and the mean error is $e = 0.1445$.

Using these coefficients, radial lens distortions for any value of r can be readily calculated.

Appendix II: Overview of Morphological Operations and Artificial Neural Networks

The grayscale dilation and erosion operations are explained by first describing their corresponding binary. Defining A and B as two sets, the binary dilation of A by B, denoted $A \oplus B$, is defined as (Gonzalez and Wood 2002)

$$A \oplus B = \left\{ z \mid \left(\hat{B}\right)_z \cap A \neq 0 \right\} \tag{II.1}$$

This is based on obtaining the reflection of B, the structuring element, about its origin and $\left(\hat{B}\right)$ shifting this reflection by z. The dilation of A by B, then, is the set of all displacements, z, such that A and B overlap at least one element. According to this interpretation, Equation II.1 may be rewritten as

$$A \oplus B = \left\{ z \mid \left[\left(\hat{B}\right)_z \cap A \right] \subseteq A \right\} \tag{II.2}$$

Figure AII.1a shows a simple set, and Figure AII.1b shows a structuring element and its reflection (the dark dot denotes the origin of the element). In this case, the structuring element and its reflection are equal because B is symmetric with respect to its origin. The dashed line in Figure AII.1c shows the original set for reference, and the solid line shows the limit beyond which any further displacements of the origin of $\hat{B}$ by z would

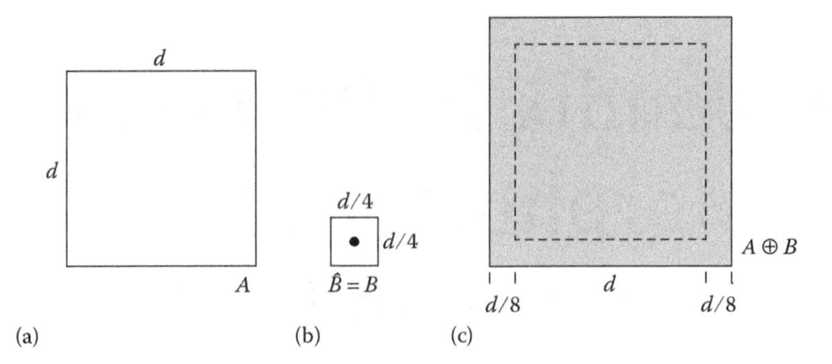

FIGURE AII.1 Binary dilation operation: (a) set A; (b) structuring; (c) dilation result. (From Gonzalez and Wood, *Digital Image Processing*, Englewood Cliffs, NJ, Prentice Hall, 2002.)

cause the intersection of $\hat{B}$ and A to be empty. Therefore, all points inside this boundary constitute the dilation of A by B.

For sets A and B, the binary erosion of A by B, denoted $A \ominus B$, is defined as

$$A \ominus B = \{z \mid (B)_z \subseteq A\} \tag{II.3}$$

This equation indicates that the erosion of A by B is the set of all points z such that B, translated by z, is contained in A. As in the dilation example, set A is shown as a dashed line for reference in Figure AII.2c. The boundary of the shaded region shows the limit beyond which further displacement of the origin of B would cause this set to cease being completely contained in A. Thus, the locus of points within this boundary (the shaded region) constitutes the erosion of A by B.

Figure AII.3a shows a binary image composed of squares of sizes 1, 3, 5, 7, 8, and 15 pixels. To remove all the squares except the large ones, we can use the erosion operation with a structuring element a size smaller than the square we want to keep. Figure AII.3b shows the result of eroding Figure AII.3a with a structuring element of size 13×13 pixels. Only portions of the largest squares remain. We can restore these three squares to their original 15×15 size by dilating them with the same structuring element used for erosion, as shown in Figure AII.3c.

The grayscale dilation and erosion operations are defined as follows. Throughout the following discussions, we deal with digital image

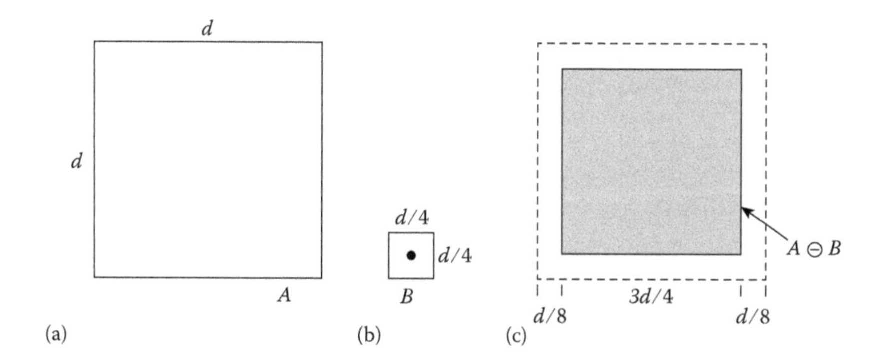

FIGURE AII.2 Binary erosion operation: (a) set A; (b) structuring; (c) erosion result. (From Gonzalez and Wood, *Digital Image Processing*, Englewood Cliffs, NJ, Prentice Hall, 2002.)

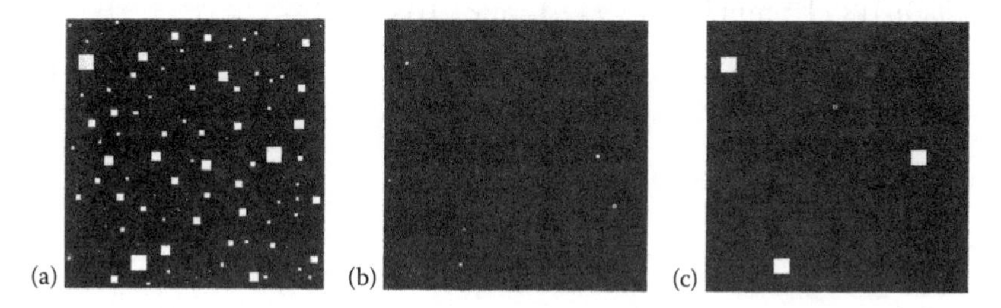

FIGURE AII.3 Binary erosion and dilation operations example: (a) original image; (b) erosion of (a); (c) dilation of (b). (From Gonzalez and Wood, *Digital Image Processing*, Englewood Cliffs, NJ, Prentice Hall, 2002.)

functions of the form $f(x, y)$ and $b(x, y)$, where $f(x, y)$ is the input image and $b(x, y)$ is a structuring element, itself a subimage function. Let Z denote the set of real integers and assume that (x, y) are integers from $Z \times Z$ and that f and b are functions for assigning a gray-level value (a real number from the set of real numbers R) to each distinct pair of coordinates (x, y). If the gray levels also are integers, Z replaces R. Grayscale dilation of f by b, denoted $f \oplus b$, is defined as

$$(f \oplus b)(s,t) = \max\{f(s-x,t-y) + b(x,y) \mid (s-x),(t-y) \in D_f; (x,y) \in D_b\} \tag{II.4}$$

where D_f and D_b are the domains of f and b, respectively. The condition that $(s-x)$ and $(t-y)$ have to be in the domain of f, and x and y have to be in the domain of b, is analogous to the condition in the definition of binary dilation as in Equation II.2, where the two sets have to overlap by at least one element.

Figure AII.4 shows a grayscale dilation example. Figure AII.4a is a simple function f, and Figure AII.4b is a structuring element b of height A. Figure AII.4c shows the structuring element b sliding by f. In Figure AII.4d, the result of dilation is shown in a solid line, and the dashed line shows the original function f for reference. There are two general effects of dilating a grayscale image: (1) if all the values of the structuring element are positive, the resulting image tends to be brighter than the original; (2) dark details are either reduced or removed, depending on how their values and shapes relate to the structuring element.

Grayscale erosion, denoted $f \ominus b$, is defined as

$$(f \ominus b)(s,t) = \min\{f(s+x,t+y) - b(x,y) \mid (s+x),(t+y) \in D_f;(x,y) \in D_b\} \tag{II.5}$$

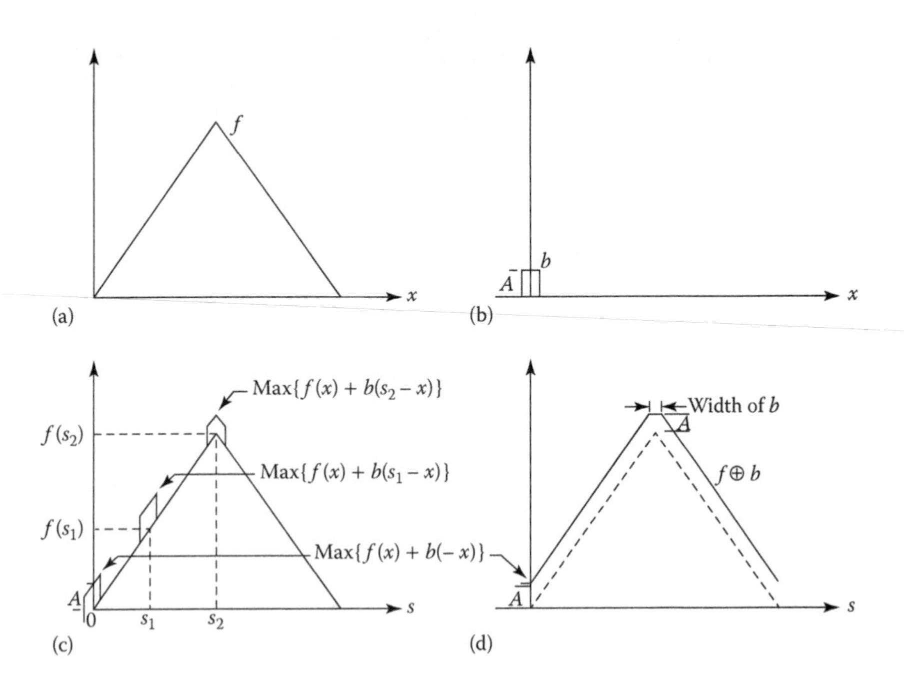

FIGURE AII.4 Grayscale dilation operation: (a) a simple function f; (b) structuring element b of height A; (c) result of dilation of sliding b past f; (d) complete result of dilation (shown solid). (From Gonzalez and Wood, *Digital Image Processing*, Englewood Cliffs, NJ, Prentice Hall, 2002.)

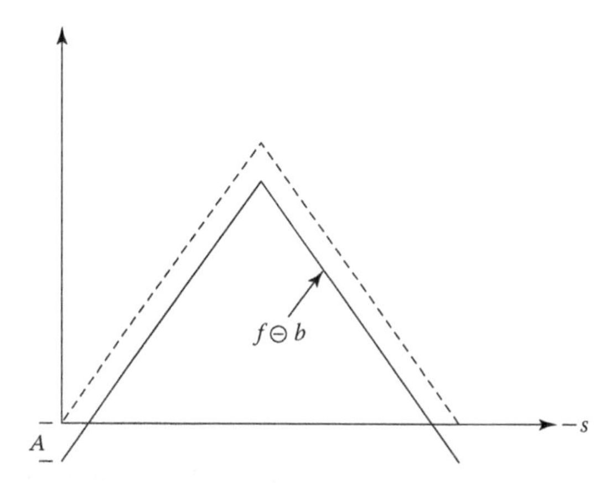

FIGURE AII.5 Grayscale erosion operation of the function f in Figure AIII.4a by the structuring element b shown in Figure AIII.4b. (From Gonzalez and Wood, *Digital Image Processing*, Englewood Cliffs, NJ, Prentice Hall, 2002.)

where D_f and D_b are the domains of f and b, respectively. The condition that $(s+x)$ and $(t+y)$ have to be in the domain of f, and x and y have to be in the domain of b, is analogous to the condition in the definition of binary erosion, as in Equation II.3, where the structuring element has to be completely contained by the set being eroded. Figure AII.5 shows the result of eroding the function f in Figure AII.4a by the structuring element b in Figure AII.4b. The result of erosion is shown in a solid line, and the dashed line shows the original function f for reference. There are two general effects of eroding a grayscale image: (1) If all the elements of the structuring are positive, the resulting image tends to be darker than the original. (2) The effect of bright detail in the original image smaller in area than the structuring element is reduced, with the degree of reduction being determined by the gray-level values surrounding the bright detail and by the shape and amplitude values of the structuring element itself.

ARTIFICIAL NEURAL NETWORKS

A Simple Neuron

An artificial neuron is a device (or computational module) with many inputs and one output, as shown in Figure AII.6 (Stergiou and Siganos 2016). The neuron has two modes of operation: training mode and using mode. In training mode, the neuron can be trained to fire (or not) for particular input patterns. In using mode, when a taught input pattern is

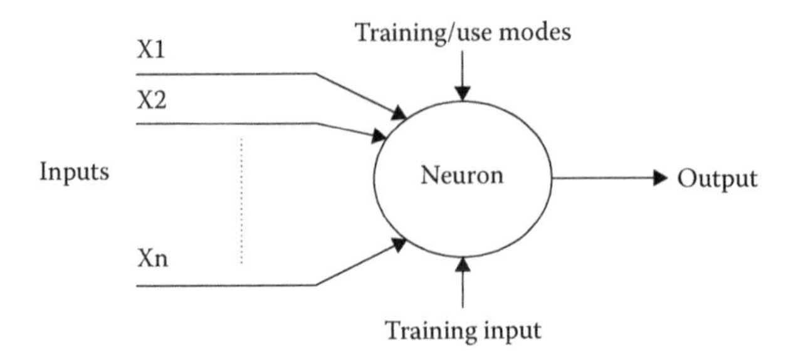

FIGURE AII.6 A simple neuron.

detected at the input, its associated output becomes the current output. If the input pattern does not belong in the taught list of input patterns, the firing rule is used to determine whether to fire or not.

Firing Rules

Firing rules are an important concept in artificial neural networks (ANNs) and account for their high flexibility. A firing rule determines how one calculates whether a neuron should fire for any input pattern. It relates to all the input patterns, not only the ones on which the node was trained.

A simple firing rule can be implemented by using the Hamming distance technique. The rule goes as follows: *Take a collection of training patterns for a node, some of which cause it to fire (the 1-taught set of patterns) and others that prevent it from doing so (the 0-taught set). Then the patterns not in the collection cause the node to fire if, on comparison, they have more input elements in common with the "nearest" pattern in the 1-taught set than with the "nearest" pattern in the 0-taught set. If there is a tie, then the pattern remains in the undefined state.*

For example, a three-input neuron is taught to output 1 when the input (X1, X2, and X3) is 111 or 101 and to output 0 when the input is 000 or 001 (as shown in Table AII.1).

As an example of the way the firing rule is applied, take the pattern 010. It differs from 000 in 1 element, from 001 in 2 elements, from 101 in

TABLE AII.1 Truth Table for a Three-Input Neuron Example

X1:	0	0	0	0	1	1	1	1
X2:	0	0	1	1	0	0	1	1
X3:	0	1	0	1	0	1	0	1
OUT:	0	0	0/1	0/1	0/1	1	0/1	1

TABLE AII.2 Truth Table for a Three-Input Neuron Example after Applying the Firing Rule

X1:	0	0	0	0	1	1	1	1
X2:	0	0	1	1	0	0	1	1
X3:	0	1	0	1	0	1	0	1
OUT:	0	0	0	0/1	0/1	1	1	1

3 elements, and from 111 in 2 elements. Therefore, the "nearest" pattern is 000, which belongs in the 0-taught set. Thus, the firing rule requires that the neuron should not fire when the input is 001. On the other hand, 011 is equally distant from two taught patterns that have different outputs and thus the output stays undefined (0/1). By applying the firing in every column, Table AII.2 can be obtained.

The difference between Tables AII.1 and AII.2 is called the *generalization of the neuron*. Therefore, the firing rule gives the neuron a sense of similarity and enables it to respond *sensibly* to patterns not seen during training.

A More Complicated Neuron

The neuron shown in Figure AII.7 is the McCulloch and Pitts model (MCP). The difference from the previous model is that the inputs are *weighted*: the effect that each input has on decision making is dependent on the weight of the particular input. The weight of an input is a number that when multiplied with the input gives the weighted input. These weighted inputs are then added together and if they exceed a preset threshold value, *T*, the neuron fires. In any other case, the neuron does not fire.

In mathematical terms, the neuron fires if and only if

$$X1W1+X2W2+X3W3+\cdots>T$$

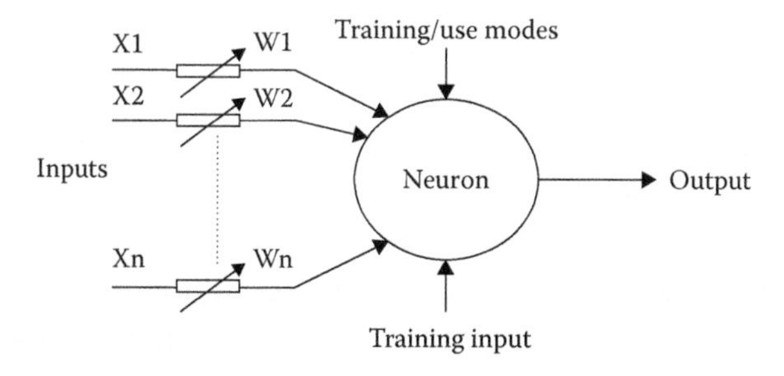

FIGURE AII.7 An MCP neuron.

The addition of input weights and of the threshold makes this neuron a very flexible and powerful one. The MCP neuron has the ability to *adapt* to a particular situation by changing its weights and/or threshold. Various algorithms exist that cause the neuron to adapt; the most used ones are the Delta rule and the back-error propagation. The former is used in feed-forward networks and the latter in feedback networks.

Feed-Forward Networks

Feed-forward ANNs allow signals to travel one way only: from input to output. There are no feedback loops; that is, the output of any layer does not affect that same layer. Feed-forward ANNs tend to be straightforward networks that associate inputs with outputs. They are extensively used in pattern recognition. This type of organization is also referred to as *bottom-up* or *top-down*.

Feedback Networks

Feedback networks can have signals traveling in both directions by introducing loops in the network. Feedback networks are very powerful and can become extremely complicated. Feedback networks are dynamic; their "state" is changing continuously until they reach an equilibrium point. They remain at the equilibrium point until the input changes and a new equilibrium needs to be found. Feedback architectures are also referred to as *interactive* or *recurrent*, although the latter term is often used to denote feedback connections in single-layer organizations.

Network Layers

The most common type of ANN consists of three groups, or layers, of units: a layer of *input* units is connected to a layer of *hidden* units, which is connected to a layer of *output* units. Here, the activity of the input units represents the raw information that is fed into the network. The activity of each hidden unit is determined by the activities of the input units and the weights on the connections between the input and the hidden units. The behavior of the output units depends on the activity of the hidden units and the weights between the hidden and output units.

This simple type of network is interesting because the hidden units are free to construct their own representations of the input. The weights between the input and hidden units determine when each hidden unit is active, and so by modifying these weights, a hidden unit can choose what it represents.

We also distinguish single-layer and multilayer architectures. The single-layer organization, in which all units are connected to one another, constitutes the most general case and is of more potential computational power than hierarchically structured multilayer organizations. In multilayer networks, units are often numbered by layer, instead of following a global numbering.

Learning Process

The memorization of patterns and the subsequent response of the network can be categorized into two general paradigms:

1. *Associative mapping*: In associative mapping, the network learns to produce a particular pattern on the set of input units whenever another particular pattern is applied on the set of input units. Associative mapping can generally be broken down into two mechanisms:

   a. *Auto-association* refers to when an input pattern is associated with itself and the states of input and output units coincide. This is used to provide pattern completion—that is, to produce a pattern whenever a portion of it or a distorted pattern is presented. In the second case, the network actually stores pairs of patterns, building an association between two sets of patterns.

   b. *Hetero-association* is related to two recall mechanisms: (i) *nearest-neighbor* recall, where the output pattern produced corresponds to the input pattern stored, which is closest to the pattern presented; and (ii) *interpolative* recall, where the output pattern is a similarity-dependent interpolation of the patterns stored corresponding to the pattern presented.

   Yet another paradigm that is a variant of associative mapping is *classification*—that is, when there is a fixed set of categories into which the input patterns are to be classified.

2. *Regularity detection*: In regularity detection, units learn to respond to particular properties of the input patterns. Whereas in associative mapping the network stores the relationships among patterns, in regularity detection the response of each unit has a particular *meaning*. This type of learning mechanism is essential for feature discovery and knowledge representation.

Every neural network possesses knowledge that is contained in the values of the connection weights. Modifying the knowledge stored in the network as a function of experience implies a learning rule for changing the values of the weights. Information is stored in the weight matrix W of a neural network. Learning is the determination of the weights. Following the way learning is performed, we can distinguish two major categories of neural networks: (1) *Fixed networks*, in which the weights cannot be changed; that is, $dW/dt = 0$. In such networks, the weights are fixed *a priori* according to the problem to solve. (2) *Adaptive networks* that are able to change their weights; that is, $dW/dt \neq 0$.

All learning methods used for adaptive neural networks can be classified into two major categories:

1. *Supervised learning*, which incorporates an external teacher, so that each output unit is told what its desired response to input signals ought to be. During the learning process, global information may be required. Paradigms of supervised learning include *error correction learning*, *reinforcement learning*, and *stochastic learning*. An important issue concerning supervised learning is the problem of error convergence—that is, the minimization of error between the desired and computed unit values. The aim is to determine a set of weights that minimizes the error. One well-known method that is common to many learning paradigms is the least mean squares (LMS) convergence.
2. *Unsupervised learning* uses no external teacher and is based on only local information. It is also referred to as *self-organization*, in the sense that it self-organizes data presented to the network and detects their emergent collective properties. Paradigms of unsupervised learning are *Hebbian learning* and *competitive learning*. The aspect of learning concerns the distinction or not of a separate phase, during which the network is trained, and a subsequent operation phase. We say that a neural network learns *offline* if the learning phase and the operation phase are distinct. A neural network learns *online* if it learns and operates at the same time. Usually, supervised learning is performed offline, whereas unsupervised learning is performed online.

Transfer Function

The behavior of an ANN depends on both the weights and the input–output function (transfer function) that is specified for the units. This function typically falls into one of three categories: (1) *linear* (or ramp), (2) *threshold*, or (3) *sigmoid*.

In linear units, the output activity is proportional to the total weighted output. For threshold units, the output is set at one of two levels, depending on whether the total input is greater than or less than some threshold value. For sigmoid units, the output varies continuously but not linearly as the input changes. Sigmoid units bear a greater resemblance to real neurons than do linear or threshold units, but all three must be considered rough approximations.

To make an ANN that performs some specific task, we must choose how the units are connected to one another and select appropriate weights for each connections. The connections determine whether it is possible for one unit to influence another. The weights specify the strength of the influence.

A three-layer network can be trained to perform a particular task by using the following procedure:

1. Present the network with training examples, which consist of a pattern of activities for the input units together with the desired pattern of activities for the output units

2. Determine how closely the actual output of the network matches the desired output

3. Change the weight of each connection so that the network produces a better approximation of the desired output

Back-Propagation Algorithm

In order to train a neural network to perform some task, the weights of each unit must be adjusted in such a way that the error between the desired output and the actual output is reduced. This process requires that the neural network compute the error derivative of the weights. In other words, it must calculate how the error changes as each weight is increased or decreased slightly. The back-propagation algorithm is the most widely used method for determining the weights.

Appendix III: Overview of the Adaptive Gaussian Mixture Model and Particle Filter

ADAPTIVE GAUSSIAN MIXTURE MODEL

Calculating Pixel Value Probability in RGB Images

Given a pixel $P(u, v)$, we use a triple vector $X_t = (x_r, x_g, x_b)^T$ to express the RGB values for P at current time t. The probability of pixel P having value X_t can be modeled by a mixture of k Gaussian distributions in the form of

$$P(X_t) = \sum_{i=1}^{k} w_{i,t} \eta(X_t, \mu_{i,t}, V_{i,t})$$

where $w_{i,t}$ is the weight for the ith Gaussian component at current time t, and η is the Gaussian density function with mean value $u_{i,t}$ and covariance matrix $V_{i,t}$. Generally, we assume the three RGB channels are independent and have the same variance so that the covariance matrix $V_{i,t}$ is equal to $I \cdot \sigma_{i,t}^2$, where I is the identity matrix and $\sigma_{i,t}$ is the standard deviation. Based on this assumption, the probability for each single channel having value x_t is defined as

$$P(x_t) = \sum_{i=1}^{k} w_{i,t} \eta(x_t, \mu_{i,t}, \sigma_{i,t}^2)$$

where the ith Gaussian density function at time t is

$$\eta\left(x_t,\mu_{i,t},\sigma_{i,t}^2\right)=\frac{1}{\sqrt{2\pi}\sigma_{i,t}}\exp\left[-\frac{\left(x_t-\mu_{i,t}\right)^2}{2\sigma_{i,t}^2}\right]$$

Adaptive Weight Function and Gaussian Parameters

The weight function for each Gaussian component is expressed as

$$w_{i,t}=(1-\lambda)w_{i,t-1}+\lambda F_{i,t}$$

where λ is the background learning rate and $F_{i,t}$ is a binary function to determine whether the input pixel matches the Gaussian distribution after being compared to a threshold ($F_{i,t}=1$ for a match and $F_{i,t}=0$ for a mismatch).

The mean and variance of the other remaining Gaussian components for time $t+1$ are also updated from the current time t in the form of

$$\mu_{i,t+1}=(1-\xi)\mu_{i,t}+\xi x_{t+1}$$

$$\sigma_{i,t+1}^2=(1-\xi)\sigma_{i,t}^2+\xi\left(x_{t+1}-\mu_{i,t+1}\right)^2 \quad \text{with} \quad \xi=\lambda\eta\left(x_{t+1}\,|\,\mu_{i,t+1},\sigma_{i,t+1}^2\right)$$

EXAMPLE OF A PARTICLE FILTER

This example shows how to use a particle filter to estimate the location of a person in 1-D space. The illustration of this example is shown in Figures AIII.1 and AIII.2.

Step 1: Initialization—Randomly generate particles in the 1-D space and assign the same weight to them.

Step 2: Weight update—Update the weight for each sample according to the measurement.

Step 3: Resample (if necessary)—If the effective sample size is not big enough, generate a new set of particles and assign even weights to them.

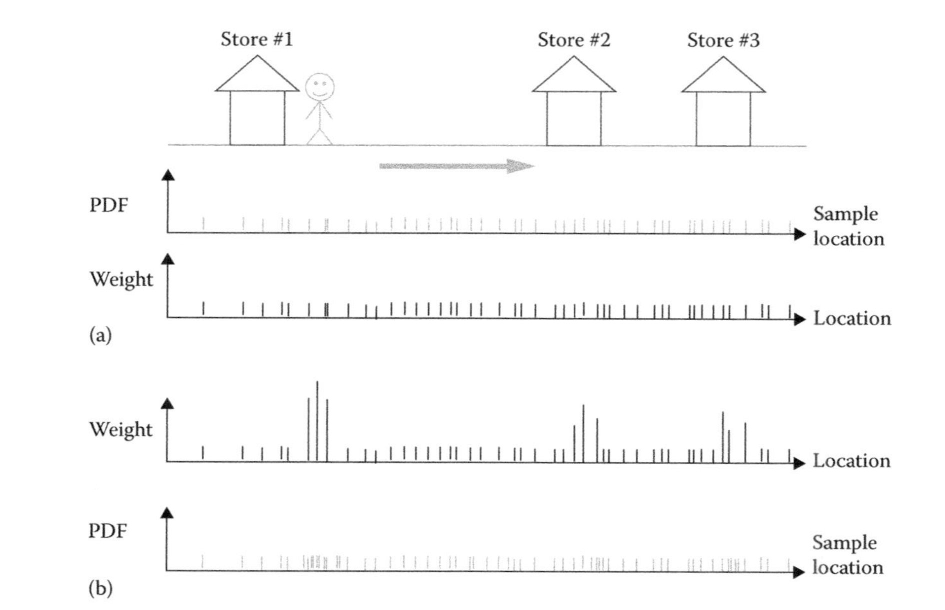

FIGURE AIII.1 Illustration of a 1-D particle filter to estimate a person's location (part 1). The thick arrow indicates the moving direction of the person. In (a), the particles (line segments) are generated at random locations and the weights are evenly assigned to them. In (b), the weights are updated according to measurement; meanwhile, the PDF for the next time $t+1$ is also updated. The new particle locations at time $t+1$ are predicted based on this PDF.

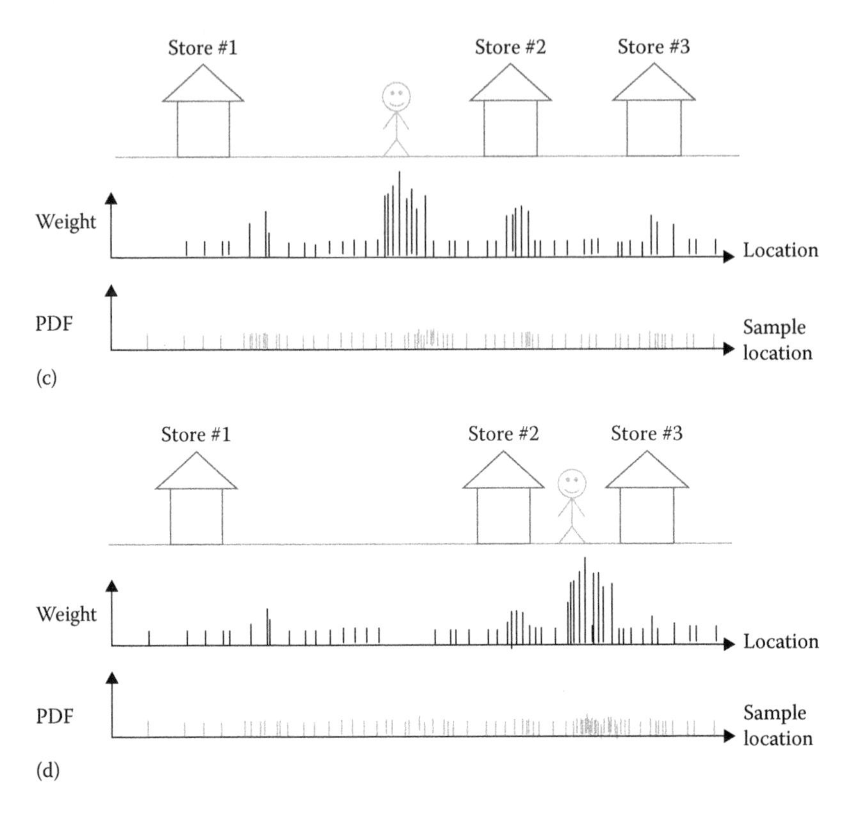

FIGURE AIII.2 Illustration of a 1-D particle filter to estimate a person's location (part 2). The PF estimations at two different times are shown in (c) and (d). As time goes on, the particles become more concentrated in the region where the person is likely to be.

Step 4: Prediction—Predict the new locations of particles according to the posterior probability density function (PDF) from the previous time $t-1$.

Step 5: Back to Step 2.

Appendix IV: Region-Matching Approaches

DETAILS OF SIFT DESCRIPTION AND EXTRACTION

Gaussian Function

In the SIFT method, the Gaussian function with variant scale σ is defined as

$$G_{x,y}(\sigma) = \frac{1}{2\pi\sigma^2} e^{-(x^2+y^2)/2\sigma^2}$$

Keypoint Candidates Filtering Procedure

The filtering procedure is applied to reject the points with low contrast or those that are poorly determined along the edge. The unstable extrema with low contrast are rejected using the Taylor expansion of the DoG function at the sample point. In order to eliminate the edge responses, we need to compare the principal curvature with its perpendicular direction. The general method is to analyze the eigenvalues of the 2×2 Hessian matrix. Equation II.1 gives the definition of the Hessian matrix:

$$H = \begin{bmatrix} \frac{\partial^2 D}{\partial x^2} & \frac{\partial^2 D}{\partial x \partial y} \\ \frac{\partial^2 D}{\partial y \partial x} & \frac{\partial^2 D}{\partial y^2} \end{bmatrix} \quad \text{(IV.1)}$$

where D represents the DoG image. Instead of computing the eigenvalues explicitly, we simply check the ratio r between the bigger magnitude eigenvalue and the smaller one according to Equation IV.2:

$$\frac{Tr(\mathrm{H})^2}{Det(\mathrm{H})} < \frac{(r+1)^2}{r} \tag{IV.2}$$

where $Tr(\mathrm{H})$ and $Det(\mathrm{H})$ are the trace and determinant of H, respectively.

SIFT Description and Extraction

Keypoint Descriptor Design

A 128-element feature vector is used to describe a keypoint. This vector is created from the 16 × 16 sample array around each keypoint. Similar to the keypoint orientation assignment, the gradient magnitude and direction are calculated for every sample point and the magnitude is weighted by a Gaussian window with a scale equal to one-half the width of Gaussian window. The 16 × 16 sample array is divided into sixteen 4 × 4 subregions. Each subregion is given an 8-bin orientation histogram covering a 360° range. The weighted orientations of the sample points are grouped into eight directions. The distribution of the orientation histogram for each subregion is visualized in an intuitive way using eight arrows. The length and the direction of the arrows represent the magnitude and orientation of the corresponding bins, respectively. To make the descriptor more robust to illumination change, some further processing steps such as filtering and normalization are added.

DETAILS OF SURF DESCRIPTION AND EXTRACTION

Integral Image

The concept of an integral image is defined in the Viola–Jones algorithm. Given an arbitrary location $P(x, y)$, the pixel value at this location in the corresponding integral image is

$$I_{\Sigma}(x, y) = \sum_{i=1}^{x} \sum_{j=1}^{y} I_{i,j}$$

where $I_{i,j}$ is the intensity of the input image.

SURF Descriptor Construction

The scale of the keypoint is determined first according to the determinant of the Hessian matrix:

$$\det\left(H_{\text{approx}}\right) = \hat{D}_{xx}\hat{D}_{yy} - \left(0.9\hat{D}_{xy}\right)^2$$

where $\hat{D}_{xx}, \hat{D}_{xy}$, and $\hat{D}_{yy}$ are the alternative box filters and 0.9 is calculated from the Frobenius norm ratio. The filter responses are further normalized with respect to the mask size so it can keep the constancy of the Frobenius norm regardless of the filter size.

Once the scale s of the keypoint is selected, a reproducible orientation is first assigned to each keypoint to make it invariant to image rotation. This stage requires the calculation of Haar wavelet responses along the x and y directions in a circular neighborhood around the keypoint. The wavelet responses are weighted with a Gaussian function centered at the keypoint. The dominant orientation of the keypoint is estimated by summing up all the horizontal and vertical responses within a sliding window that covers an angle of 60°.

After the orientation for each keypoint is determined, a square region is then generated at the center of the keypoint with size $20s$ and oriented along the selected orientation. The x and y axes for each region are also rotated accordingly. To design the descriptor, the square region is split into 4×4 subregions and every subregion is sampled 5×5 times. The Haar wavelet responses in the x and y directions are calculated within each subregion, respectively. By adding up all the wavelet responses and their absolute values at the sample points in the subregion, we can get a 4D feature vector v:

$$v = \left(\sum d_x, \sum d_y, \sum |d_x|, \sum |d_y|\right)$$

In this equation, d_x and d_y are the Haar wavelet responses for both directions. Taking account of all the 4×4 subregions, we will have a 64-dimensional descriptor vector V:

$$V = (v_1, v_2, \ldots, v_i, \ldots, v_{16})$$

An alternative version called SURF-128 extends the number of descriptor entries to 128 by introducing similar features. In SURF-128, Σd_x and $\Sigma|d_x|$ are separately computed under $d_y < 0$ and $d_y \geq 0$, and a similar operation is applied to Σd_y and $\Sigma|d_y|$.

DETAILS OF ORB DESCRIPTION AND EXTRACTION

Steered BRIEF

The location pairs (x, y) are firstly rotated by the patch orientation θ and a steered version of BRIEF $g_n(p, \theta)$ is constructed based on the new location pairs:

$$g_n(p,\theta) = f_n(p) \mid (\tilde{x}_i, \tilde{y}_i) \in \tilde{S}$$

where $\tilde{S}$ is the rotated location pair matrix.

RANSAC Paradigm and Pseudocode

The *random sample consensus* (RANSAC) paradigm consists of the following steps:

Step 1: Randomly select a subset $S_1[n]$ from input points $P[N]$.

Step 2: Compute the model M from $S_1[n]$.

Step 3: Find inliers and outliers according to M and a reprojection threshold.

Step 4: Recompute model M' from all the inliers $S_1^*[m]$ if m is big enough; if not, repeat Step 1.

The initial subset $S_1[n]$ is the minimum number of required points to initially instantiate the model M. The number of iterative times is predefined to satisfy the possibility of finding the largest consensus set. The final estimated model M is from this largest consensus set. The pseudocode for the RANSAC algorithm is as follows:

```
1. Set P[N]
2. Randomly select S_1[n]
3. Set T = 1
4. Instantiate model M from S_1[n]
5. While T < T_max + 1, do
6.      Determine S_1^*[m] using M
7.      If m > threshold t, then
8.          Update M based on S_1^*[m]
9.      Else
10.         Randomly select S_2[n]
11.         Instantiate model M from S_2[n]
12.     End if
13.     T = T + 1
14. End while
```

Index

H

I

K

L